Social Communication Difficulties

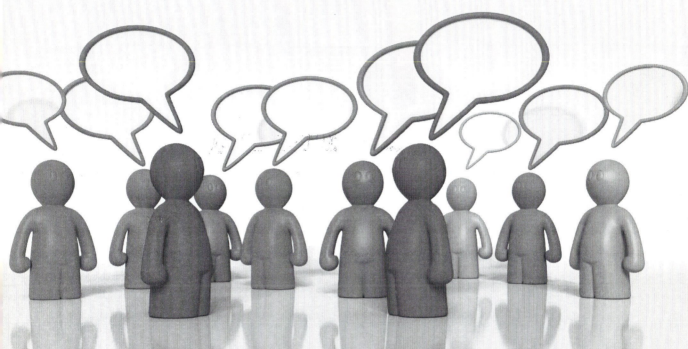

Resource Pack

Lucy Prosser, Nicola Cole, Sally Farrow, Jenny Hinton, Margaret Irons, Ann Pugmire, Emily Rackstraw, Vijaya Sudra, Caroline Sutton and Gilly Williams

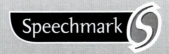
Speechmark

KH

Published by

Speechmark Publishing Ltd, Sunningdale House, 43 Caldecotte Lake Drive, Milton Keynes MK7 8LF,
United Kingdom
Tel: +44 (0)1908 277177   Fax: +44 (0)1908 278297
www.speechmark.net

002-5734 Printed in the United Kingdom by CMP (uk) Limited

British Library Cataloguing in Publication Data
A catalogue record for this book is available from the British Library.

ISBN 978 0 86388 820 5

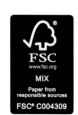

4 / 9 / 18

Contents

Introduction

This Social Communication Difficulties Resource Pack was devised by members of the speech and language therapy team in Portsmouth City teaching Primary Care Trust (PCT). It was intended to be used primarily by speech and language therapists to help with identification and assessment of social communication difficulties and to provide ideas for intervention strategies. During piloting of the resource, we became aware that other professionals, such as colleagues in education, felt that it would be a useful resource in their own teams to support and guide discussion with parents of children with social communication difficulties.

Social communication skills are the set of skills required for social purposes and involve both verbal and non-verbal communication. People need this complex set of skills in order to function in structured environments, such as school or work, as well as in relationships with family and friends. Social communication difficulties can manifest in number of different ways and at different stages of development. They can be associated with, but are not exclusive to, autism spectrum disorders.

Children seen by speech and language therapists in clinic, education setting or at home can present with a range of difficulties with social communication. In an attempt to clarify the range of difficulties, we devised an Areas and Features of Social Communication Difficulties chart (see Figure 1, page 3) that breaks down social communication difficulties into the four key areas: language, conversation skills, social skills and selecting and organising information. These key areas are then sub-divided into more detailed features of social communication difficulties. The decision to categorise the features in this way is in recognition of the varying presentations of children with social communication difficulties. The chart is intended to be used to guide assessment of children with social communication difficulties and assist with illustrating an individual child's profile when discussing their strengths and needs with a staff member and/or a carer and to guide the reader to the relevant handout(s).

Following the development of this chart, we created a set of photocopiable handouts which address each feature identified in the flowchart. Each handout provides a description of a particular social communication difficulty, examples of how this might present in children, and a list of practical suggestions for teaching the specific skills required.   However, for certain features it has been necessary to break these down into more discrete skills. For example, 'conversation skills' have been broken down into starting, maintaining, joining and ending conversations. In addition, the handouts have been devised to cover developmental levels and are referred to as early or later skills rather than developmental ages.

The handouts are intended to be a starting point for discussion with education staff and/or carers. It is recommended that they form part of a wider discussion rather than be used as a stand-alone resource. That is, it is important for the professional using the resource to explain in greater detail how to carry out the activities or to add alternative activities that may be more appropriate to an individual child.

Where necessary short references are included in individual handouts. The bibliography at the end of the pack includes these references alongside other publications which the user might find helpful as sources of further information. A glossary explains particular terms that are referred to within the pack.

With thanks to Catherine Fisher for her original thoughts and input.

Figure 1 Areas and features of social communication difficulties

SOCIAL COMMUNICATION DIFFICULTIES

LANGUAGE

Comprehension
- Understanding of non-literal language
- Following instructions
- Abstract vocabulary
- Verbal reasoning

Expression

Functions:
- Gaining attention
- Requesting (objects / actions)
- Rejecting
- Social: greeting
- Commenting
- Questioning
- Asking for help

Disordered Features:
- Unusual language
- Stereotyped language – overuse of adult-like phrases
- Language produced from learned chunks rather then used flexibly
- Echolalia – repeating back what has been heard
- Repetitive questioning

CONVERSATION SKILLS

Verbal
- Starting a conversation
- Interrupting and joining conversations
- Keeping a conversation going
- Ending a conversation
- Repairing

Non-Verbal
- Eye contact
- Turn-taking
- Facial expression
- Body language
- Proximity (personal space)
- Intonation
- Gesture

SOCIAL SKILLS

Social Interaction
- Emotional understanding
- Interactive play
- Sharing
- Negotiation and compromise
- Friendship skills

Social context
- Adapting style of communication to different social contexts

Understanding Intentions
- Bullying
- Facts/lies/ Opinions
- Humour

SELECTING AND ORGANISING INFORMATION
- Understanding of listener needs (Pre-suppositional knowledge)
- Narrative skills
- Sequencing of ideas inc: prediction

Speechmark

Language

Comprehension

Expression

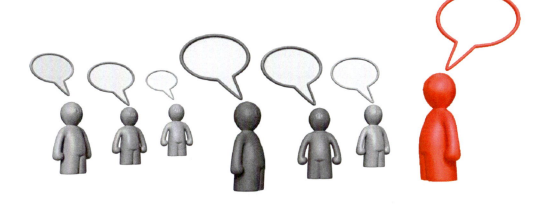

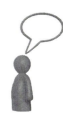

Comprehension

What do we mean by non-literal language?

When we talk, we frequently use 'non-literal' language in which what we mean may not be exactly what we are saying. Examples of non-literal language include:

- idioms (eg 'I've got butterflies in my stomach', 'pull your socks up')

- use of similes/metaphors (eg 'hair like spun gold', 'he is a sly fox')

- irony and sarcasm (eg 'Now I've broken my television, that's just great')

- lies or white lies.

Children who have difficulty understanding non-literal language:

- have particular difficulty understanding this sort of language because they interpret language very literally – they may think someone actually has butterflies in their stomach or actually go to pull their socks up when these idioms are used

- find it difficult to think abstractly and to generalise their learning

- find it difficult to think of the underlying meaning – that is, that 'pull your socks up' actually means 'try harder'

- may have difficulties reading facial expressions or interpreting tone of voice and may therefore not detect irony or sarcasm and find it difficult to tell whether people are lying

- may respond inappropriately to what you have said or ignore you if they have not understood – rather than rudeness, this is often a coping mechanism or because they don't know how to ask for clarification

- may have difficulties understanding implied meaning – for example, when someone says 'You're being noisy' they may not understand that this implies that the speaker would like them to be quieter.

  Speechmark

Ways to help children who have difficulty understanding 'non-literal' language

- Try to avoid using non-literal language wherever possible and encourage those working with the child also to be aware of using this sort of language. It is surprising how much non-literal language we use in day-to-day conversation without realising it.

- Give instructions that are short and to the point. For example, say 'Martin, close the window please' rather than 'It's very chilly in here', hoping that the child understands your implied meaning; or 'Can you close the window?', to which the child will probably be thinking 'Yes, I can', but may not realise that you actually want him to.

- If you do use an idiom or sarcasm, try to explain it (eg 'I've got butterflies in my stomach … that's what we say when we're nervous about something'). Check later to see whether the child has remembered the meaning. Ask them, 'I said I had butterflies in my stomach. What does "butterflies in your stomach" mean?' The meaning of idioms may need to be taught as it is difficult for these children to infer a meaning.

- If someone else uses non-literal language, it may be useful to provide a literal translation. For example, if another child says 'Get off my back', you could say, 'Charlotte wants to be left alone.'

- With older children, it may be useful to discuss similes, metaphors and idioms. For instance, using 'his brain is like a computer' as an example, you could discuss ways in which the brain is similar and dissimilar to a computer so that the children can start to understand why that description was used.

- Encourage the child to ask if they are unsure what you mean. It may be useful to keep a record of new idioms learned.

Speechmark

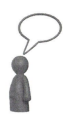

Comprehension

HOW TO SUPPORT CHILDREN WHO HAVE DIFFICULTY FOLLOWING INSTRUCTIONS

1b

Why is it important to be able to follow instructions?

The ability to follow instructions is an important skill in a variety of social situations and settings throughout life (family life, education, recreation). It enables us to carry out tasks and activities, learn new skills, work together cooperatively and conform to social rules and expectations.

Young children start to follow simple instructions at an early age, making use of situational and visual cues to support their understanding. As they become older and their understanding of spoken language develops, they also begin to develop the ability to understand and follow lengthy, more complex spoken instructions.

Children who have difficulty following instructions

Some children may show no apparent interest in instructions or may watch others in order to support their understanding. Some are better at following instructions in a one-to-one situation than in group situations.

A child's inability to follow instructions may be due to:

- difficulty with attention or concentration

- difficulty remembering and/or understanding all the instructions they have been given

- a tendency to 'switch off' or become disruptive if they are feeling overloaded or overwhelmed as a result of too much information

- difficulty understanding ambiguous language – for example, idioms (eg 'pull your socks up'), sarcasm, jokes and verbal absurdity – and a tendency to understand literally

- not realising that instructions include them, when instructions are given to the whole group (eg class instructions)

- fixed ideas about how things should be done, so that the child is unable to follow instructions from others

- no interest in following instructions, unless related to their own interests and obsessions.

Ways to support children in following instructions

- Reduce background noise as much as possible.

- Gain attention – for example, say the child's name and raise your hand or say their name and use a 'Listen' visual cue card (see Glossary).

- Speak slowly and use pauses to allow the child more time to process the information.

- Give straightforward information in short amounts (ie 'chunk information').

- Check that the child has understood what has been said.

- Repeat spoken information, using the same wording. If misunderstanding continues, consider simplifying your vocabulary or use of grammar.

- Teach and encourage requests for repetition or clarification.

- Avoid the use of idioms, sarcasm and jokes; if you do use these, explain them as you go.

- Use specific praise (see Glossary) for good listening; also use a reward chart (see Glossary).

- Play listening games, such as 'Simon Says', or games in which the child has to listen for their name or for 'Go' before they have a turn at something.

- Provide visual support (eg a visual timetable, a visual schedule, visual cue cards, pointing, gesture, photos, pictures, signs, symbols, diagrams, written lists of key points) or words, if appropriate, and worked examples (eg numeracy).

You should always take responsibility for the way in which your instructions are phrased and presented.

Speechmark

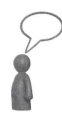

Comprehension

What do we mean by abstract vocabulary?

The term 'abstract vocabulary' is used to describe words that do not have a direct relationship to an object and will therefore be difficult to picture in one's mind. Abstract words often describe the relationship between things; they are sometimes referred to as 'language concepts' and include the vocabulary of:

- time (again, now, after, soon, early, etc)

- number and quantity (all, some, none, many, few, whole, etc)

- size (big, little, full, tall, etc)

- position (in, on, off, near, below, etc)

- attributes (noisy, good, pretty, hard, soft, colours, etc).

Children who have difficulty understanding abstract vocabulary

Children with language and social communication disorders often have difficulty learning and remembering these types of words and may need to have them specifically taught. Difficulty in understanding abstract language can result in difficulties in following instructions and in progressing in many curriculum subjects (particularly maths and science).

Children develop understanding of language concepts at different stages (eg in typical development, 'big'/'little' and 'in'/'on' at 2 years, colours at 3 years, 'in front'/'behind' at 3 years 6 months). Sometimes children can be developing concrete vocabulary well, but their development of abstract vocabulary and concepts may be uneven or characterised by specific gaps.

Ways to support development of understanding abstract vocabulary

- Teach new words one at a time and relate them only to words the child already understands (eg teach 'on' and contrast it with 'not on' rather than teach 'on' and 'off' at the same time).

- Teach abstract vocabulary in developmental order (eg you would not teach the word 'less' if the child did not understand the concept of 'all').

- Encourage the child to experience a word you are teaching (eg placing themselves 'on' and 'under' objects) – if the child can 'do' the word, they are more likely to remember it.

- Use objects to demonstrate what words mean.

- Use pictures or symbols to represent words.

- Words should be taught with a lot of repetition – revisit a word in as many different contexts as possible (eg when teaching 'on', a sticker could be placed 'on' the wall or 'on' the teacher's head and the computer or light can be turned 'on').

- Use sorting and matching to teach colour and texture.

- Teaching should be slow and careful; these are difficult words to grasp and extending too quickly into different contexts will confuse a child.

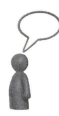

Comprehension

WORKSHEET 1D

What are verbal reasoning skills?

Verbal reasoning incorporates the skills of inference, problem solving, prediction, deduction, understanding implied meaning, understanding metaphor and analogies, applying one's own experiences, using context and understanding cause–effect relationships. Although children with verbal reasoning difficulties may have a good understanding of the actual words they hear and the pictures and scenarios they see, it is the 'reading between the lines' (the ability to guess or predict information that is not actually given) that causes their difficulties. Such difficulties are likely to be ongoing, but teaching the children strategies for seeking clarification of meaning or different ways to find information can help.

Children with verbal reasoning difficulties:

- find it hard to cope with there being more than one potential answer to a problem, and therefore find it difficult to generate or accept alternative solutions

- have difficulties with the concept of 'guessing' (they either know something or they do not know it)

- find it difficult to make connections between pieces of information (verbal or visual)

- can be anxious about being 'wrong', which may lead to a refusal to offer ideas

- may have a restricted general knowledge of the world, as a result of their focus on specific interests, which can result in difficulties with inference

- may struggle to see things from another person's point of view, and therefore to predict feelings, reactions, and so on, due to difficulties with theory of mind (see Glossary).

Ways to help children with verbal reasoning difficulties

💬 If misunderstanding occurs, be explicit in your explanation of what was meant and why the breakdown in communication occurred.

💬 Teach about categories and the similarities and differences between things (eg bananas and apples are both fruit, but they are different shapes and one is yellow and the other green or red; then go on to teach about metaphors and analogies).

💬 Develop an understanding of cause–effect relationships and problem solving by using sequence pictures, stories or DVDs to explore solutions to problems, generate alternative outcomes and predict consequences.

💬 Teach that making mistakes is OK and that there may not be a 'right' and a 'wrong'. Give specific praise (see Glossary) for the generation of different solutions or consequences.

💬 Consider published programmes, such as *Think It: Say It* (Martin, 1990), *Think About It* (Rippon, 2005) and *Problem Solving Activities* (Gaetano, 1996).

💬 Encourage children to think about their own experiences in relation to the task and to apply anything they may have learned from these.

💬 Teach children how to identify the key elements that provide 'unspoken' information (eg the look on someone's face, the context, etc).

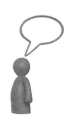

Expression

WORKSHEET 2A

What do we mean by 'the functions of language'?

We use language for a variety of different functions – for example, to get a person's **attention**, to **greet** them, to **comment** on things happening around us, to **request** things that we want or to **say 'no'** to things we don't want. We can also ask for **help**. As we get older, we develop better and more appropriate ways to use language. However, children with social communication difficulties may find these skills difficult to learn. This can impact on the way they communicate with and respond to other people.

Children in the early stages of development who have difficulty using language for a range of functions may:

- not show awareness of other people (appear to be in their own world)

- find it difficult to get another person's attention (ie to initiate)

- find it difficult to use words, signs or pictures to name things and to make comments

- find it difficult to ask for things that they want or to ask for help

- be frustrated by their inability to communicate their needs, which can lead to a range of behaviours (eg tantrums, opting out, physical and/or verbal outbursts)

- can be difficult to engage or appear passive.

Ways to encourage a child to gain attention in the early stages

Young children who have difficulty gaining attention can be helped in the following ways:

💬 Respond with a reward (a big smile, praise, positive comment) when the child looks towards you or makes eye contact.

💬 Play 'Ready, Steady, Go' games and wait for the child to look at you before you do the action (eg blow bubbles or push the car).

💬 If a child tends to gain attention by crying or shouting, model appropriate ways to gain attention (eg using a person's name or saying 'excuse me').

💬 Reward appropriate attempts to gain your attention with lots of positive feedback, so that the child wants to do it again.

💬 When playing with a toy, wait until the child looks at you before activating it.

💬 Encourage the child to point to or look at things in order to make choices – keep the item to yourself until they look at you or make a noise or say a word.

💬 Put some favourite toys out of reach and when the child indicates that they want the toy, model how to point to it and then give them the toy.

💬 Children who have significant difficulties with gaining attention may benefit from *The Picture Exchange Communication System* (PECS) approach (Frost & Bondy, 2002). Your speech and language therapist will be able to advise whether this is appropriate.

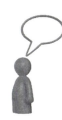

Expression

WORKSHEET 2B

What do we mean by 'the functions of language'?

We use language for a variety of different functions – for example: to get a person's **attention**, to **greet** them, to **comment** on things happening around us, to **request** things that we want or to **say 'no'** to things we don't want. We can also ask for **help**. As we get older, we develop better and more appropriate ways to use language. However, children with social communication difficulties may find these skills difficult to learn. This can impact on the way they communicate with and respond to other people.

Children in the later stages of development who have difficulty using language for different functions may:

- struggle to get other people's attention appropriately

- not respond as expected when greeted and may be unsure of how to greet others

- have difficulty asking and answering questions effectively

- struggle to talk about events or activities: they can find it hard to process, plan and sequence language, which can mean that the listener may have difficulty following their narrative

- find it difficult to give the listener the right amount of information about an event (ie they give either too little or too much)

- have difficulty using language for more sophisticated purposes, such as humour, negotiation, explanation and reasoning

- not know how to ask for clarification and help

- find it difficult to express their feelings and emotions.

Speechmark

Ways to encourage a child to gain attention in the later stages

- Raise awareness of the ways in which the child is currently attracting attention (eg shouting out in class) and discuss how appropriate or inappropriate these may be.

- Discuss different ways of gaining attention in different settings.

- Role play a range of different situations to discover whether and when certain strategies are suitable (eg shouting out to gain attention may be useful on the football pitch).

- Set targets jointly with the child that are realistic (eg 'I will put up my hand and wait when I want to talk to the teacher during the next 5 minutes').

- Use visual prompts and cue cards (see Glossary) to remind the child of useful strategies for gaining attention (eg a picture of a child putting up their hand, which you can show the child if they call out).

- Use Social Stories™ (Gray, 2001) to help prompt the child to remember the strategies they are trying and the reasons behind them.

- Use reward systems and specific praise (see Glossary) to motivate the child to use appropriate behaviours.

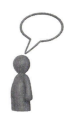

Expression

WORKSHEET 2C

What do we mean by 'the functions of language'?

We use language for a variety of different functions – for example, to get a person's **attention**, to **greet** them, to **comment** on things happening around us, to **request** things that we want or to **say** '**no**' to things we don't want. We can also ask for help. As we get older, we develop better and more appropriate ways to use language. However, children with social communication difficulties may find these skills difficult to learn. This can impact on the way they communicate with and respond to other people.

Requesting allows us to make our needs known. At an early level, a child may wish to request food items, toys or activities and, later on, help, clarification or interaction with others. The skills required are both verbal and non-verbal (eg eye gaze, pointing).

Children who have difficulty making requests:

• may appear very passive and there can be a tendency for adults to anticipate their needs, which can reinforce this passive behaviour

• may be able to gain attention, but then find it difficult to communicate what they want

• often have difficulty making choices, which is a supporting skill to initiating a request.

Ways to help children who have difficulty requesting

- Adults should create opportunities for children to request by offering choices (eg choice of clothes to wear, toys to play with, snack items to eat). Do this by holding up the real objects and asking 'Which one do you want?' Even if you think you know what they want, still offer choices and try not to anticipate their needs.

- Children can be encouraged to request an item (eg food, drink, a toy), an activity (eg singing, cuddle, water play) or a place (eg a park or garden, or home) using a variety of means, including pointing (using hands or eye pointing), gestures, Makaton signs (see Glossary), pictures and words. Your speech and language therapist will be able to advise on which methods will be most appropriate for each child.

- Create opportunities for the child to request by 'sabotage' (see Glossary) (eg put on only one shoe, put a toy out of their reach, remove pieces from a puzzle, give them paper and no crayons). Wait for them to gain your attention and then model an appropriate request (eg say 'shoe' and make the sign for shoe).

- Children need to hear a word or see a sign many, many times before they are able to use it to request spontaneously. Regularly give a clear model of the word and/or the sign (eg by saying 'drink' and doing the sign for drink every time the child has a drink).

- An early request to teach a child is 'more', using the Makaton sign, a picture or the spoken word. Choose activities the child is highly motivated by (eg bubbles or a favourite food). Give them one bit of food or one blow of the bubbles and then, if they want more, show them the sign for 'more' alongside saying the word. Initially, they may need hand-over-hand assistance with the signing. After a couple of attempts, provide an opportunity for the child to request spontaneously and give cues (eg by leaning forward with an anticipatory facial expression and giving the first sound of the word or using a sign until the child is requesting spontaneously). Practise using a variety of motivators and at different times during the day to help with generalisation.

- Children who do not request or initiate at all may benefit from a structured visual approach. Your speech and language therapist may recommend such approaches as *The Picture Exchange Communication System* (Frost & Bondy, 2002).

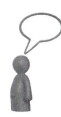

Expression

WORKSHEET 2D

What do we mean by 'the functions of language'?

We use language for a variety of different functions – for example, to get a person's **attention**, to **greet** them, to **comment** on things happening around us, to **request** things that we want or to **say 'no'** to things we don't want. We can also ask for **help**. As we get older, we develop better and more appropriate ways to use language. However, children with social communication difficulties may find these skills difficult to learn. This can impact on the way they communicate with and respond to other people.

Being able to say 'no' to something allows us to have some control over our environment and the things we are asked to do. There are many different ways to reject or refuse something and how we do this will depend on the social situation. It will be influenced by who we are talking to, the setting we are in and what we are actually being offered, (the way we might say 'no' to someone trying to take something we own is very different from how we would say 'no' to the offer of a drink at a friend's house).

Children who have difficulty using language for different functions may:

- struggle to get other people's attention appropriately

- not respond as expected when greeted and may be unsure of how to greet others

- have difficulty asking and answering questions effectively

- struggle to talk about events or activities: they can find it hard to process, plan and sequence language, which can mean that the listener may have difficulty following their narrative

- find it difficult to give the listener the right amount of information about an event (ie they give either too little too much)

- have difficulty using language for more sophisticated purposes, such as humour, negotiation, explanation and reasoning

- not know how to ask for clarification and help

- find it difficult to express their feelings and emotions.

Speechmark

WORKSHEET 2D

Ways to encourage appropriate rejection of items, actions or people

Children with social communication difficulties can reject things by using many different behaviours and have difficulties with expressing verbally that they don't want something. High levels of anxiety, coupled with sensory issues, can result in children with social communication difficulties rejecting many things that others would not. It is important that adults involved recognise the communicative intent behind the behaviour and deal with it appropriately (eg if a child is hitting, is this to say 'no', to make contact with a peer, to gain attention or to say they want more of something?).

- Play sorting games using pictures or objects to encourage a child to develop an understanding of what they like and dislike (eg food, television programmes, places).

- Expand the activity in the point above to teach a child how to express these likes and dislikes by modelling appropriate verbal and non-verbal responses.

- Rejection can be expressed in a number of different ways (eg non-verbally through facial expression, body posture, sign and gesture, and verbally through words or phrases): Choosing the most appropriate ways of rejecting something will depend on the individual child's stage of development.

- Model a more appropriate form of rejection (eg if a child screeches, model a more appropriate response, such as 'No, thank you').

- Use role play to demonstrate and practise the effectiveness and range of different ways to reject things.

Speechmark

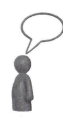

Expression

What do we mean by 'the functions of language'?

We use language for a variety of different functions – for example, to get a person's **attention**, to **greet** them, to **comment** on things happening around us, to **request** things that we want or to **say** 'no' to things we don't want. We can also ask for **help**. As we get older, we develop better and more appropriate ways to use language. However, children with social communication difficulties may find these skills difficult to learn. This can impact on the way they communicate with and respond to other people.

Children in the early stages of development who have difficulty using language for a range of functions may:

- not show awareness of other people (appear to be in their own world)

- find it difficult to get another person's attention (ie to initiate)

- find it difficult to use words, signs or pictures to name things and to make comments

- find it difficult to ask for things that they want or to ask for help

- be frustrated by their inability to communicate their needs, which can lead to a range of behaviours (eg tantrums, opting out, physical and/or verbal outbursts)

- can be difficult to engage or appear passive.

Ways to encourage the use of language for greetings in the early stages

- Play 'Peek-a-Boo' games: hide your eyes with your hands or a cloth and uncover your face, saying 'Hello'.

- Use a 'feely' bag with soft toys, animals or vehicles (follow the child's interests), take turns to take out a toy and model a greeting as you do so, such as 'Hello, Teddy', 'Hello, car'. Similarly, when you put toys away, model 'Bye, Teddy', 'Bye, car'.

- Make the most of everyday social situations (eg if someone says 'Hello' to the child, draw the child's attention to this and encourage them to say 'Hello' back).

- In circle time (see Glossary), encourage children to greet each other (eg 'Ashley, go and say "Hello" to Kieran').

- Sing songs that incorporate greetings – use a 'hello' song and a 'goodbye' song consistently at the beginning and end of each session.

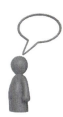

Expression

What do we mean by 'the functions of language'?

We use language for a variety of different functions – for example, to get a person's **attention**, to **greet** them, to **comment** on things happening around us, to **request** things that we want or to **say** 'no' to things we don't want. We can also ask for **help**. As we get older, we develop better and more appropriate ways to use language. However, children with social communication difficulties may find these skills difficult to learn. This can impact on the way they communicate with and respond to other people.

Children in the later stages of development who have difficulty using language for a range of functions may:

- struggle to get other people's attention appropriately

- not respond as expected when greeted and may be unsure of how to greet others

- have difficulty asking and answering questions effectively

- struggle to talk about events or activities: they can find it hard to process, plan and sequence language, which can mean that the listener may have difficulty following their narrative

- find it difficult to give the listener the right amount of information about an event (ie they give either too little or too much)

- have difficulty using language for more sophisticated purposes, such as humour, negotiation, explanation and reasoning

- not know how to ask for clarification and help

- find it difficult to express their feelings and emotions.

WORKSHEET 2F

Ways to encourage the use of language for greetings in the later stages

- Raise the child's awareness of the range of ways in which language is used to greet people. Talk about non-verbal (eg raising eyebrows, smiling) as well as verbal ('Hi', 'Hey', 'Hello', etc) forms of greeting.

- Discuss how different greeting styles are appropriate for different people and/or different situations (eg the child would greet their teacher in a different way from greeting a friend).

- Use role play and/or look at videos or DVDs to observe different kinds of greeting.

- Use a reward system and specific praise (see Glossary) to motivate the child to use appropriate greetings.

- Use visual prompts (see Glossary) or Social Stories™ (Gray, 2001) to help remind the child of strategies they could use.

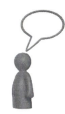

Expression

What do we mean by 'the functions of language'?

We use language for a variety of different functions – for example, to get a person's **attention**, to **greet** them, to **comment** on things happening around us, to **request** things that we want or to **say** 'no' to things we don't want. We can also ask for **help**. As we get older, we develop better and more appropriate ways to use language. However, children with social communication difficulties may find these skills difficult to learn. This can impact on the way they communicate with and respond to other people.

Children who have difficulty using language for a range of functions may:

- not show awareness of other people (appear to be in their own world)

- find it difficult to get another person's attention (ie to initiate)

- find it difficult to use words, signs or pictures to name things and to make comments

- find it difficult to ask for things that they want or to ask for help

- be frustrated by their inability to communicate their needs, which can lead to a range of behaviours (eg tantrums, opting out, physical and/or verbal outbursts)

- can be difficult to engage or appear passive.

Ways to encourage the use of commenting

Model or say (and sign if appropriate) words to describe what the child is playing with, what they are looking at or what they can hear. Children need to hear a word and/or see a sign many times before they will use it spontaneously, so a lot of repetition is necessary.

Leave a pause when pointing things out in order to encourage the child to join in (eg 'Oh look, it's a …').

Create opportunities for the child to comment by looking at books and describing what you see, or naming toys as you tidy up or get toys out to play with.

Model phrases such as 'I see …' or 'I hear …' to encourage the child to comment on or label things around them (like an 'I Spy' game without the guessing element).

Speechmark

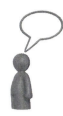

Expression

WORKSHEET 2H

What do we mean by 'the functions of language'?

We use language for a variety of different functions – for example, to get a person's **attention**, to **greet** them, to **comment** on things happening around us, to **request** things that we want or to **say 'no'** to things we don't want. We can also ask for **help**. We use **questions** to learn more about the people and the world around us. As we get older, we develop better and more appropriate ways to use language. However, children with social communication difficulties may find these skills difficult to learn. This can impact on the way they communicate with and respond to other people.

Children who have difficulty asking and answering questions may:

• not appear to be interested in what is being talked about

• appear rude or offensive by asking inappropriate questions

• ask too many questions and disrupt the flow of conversation

• not seek clarification when they have misunderstood something

• find it hard to initiate and sustain a conversation

• have limited understanding of things around them because they do not always ask for information or question what they have been told.

Speechmark

Children may find some of the following skills difficult	Ways to encourage these skills
Asking questions	Model asking simple questions (who/where/what). Play barrier games (see Glossary). Play 'Who am I?' or twenty-question type games with familiar people and objects. Carry out narrative skills activities (see Glossary) around who, where, what happened and when, using visual prompts and cue cards (see Glossary).
Asking the right number of questions	Model appropriate use of questions (eg gaining attention first, giving time to respond, asking one question at a time). If a question is asked repeatedly, be consistent in only responding the first time it is asked – avoid responding to later repetitions of the same question.
Asking/replying to 'social questions'	Model 'social questions' (eg 'How are you?', 'What are you doing?', 'Are you having a nice time?', etc) and encourage the child to use these. Make them part of everyday social interactions with adults and other children and praise attempts to use this higher level of questioning.

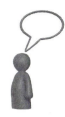

Expression

WORKSHEET 2I

What do we mean by 'the functions of language'?

We use language for a variety of different functions – for example, to get a person's **attention**, to **greet** them, to **comment** on things happening around us, to **request** things that we want or to **say 'no'** to things we don't want. We can also ask for **help**. As we get older, we develop better and more appropriate ways to use language. However, children with social communication difficulties may find these skills difficult to learn. This can impact on the way they communicate with and respond to other people.

Children in the early stages of development who have difficulty using language for a range of functions may:

- not show awareness of other people (appear to be in their own world)

- find it difficult to get another person's attention (ie to initiate)

- find it difficult to use words, signs or pictures to name things and to make comments

- find it difficult to ask for things that they want or to ask for help

- be frustrated by their inability to communicate their needs, which lead to a range of behaviours (eg tantrums, opting out, physical and/or verbal outbursts)

- can be difficult to engage or appear passive.

Ways to encourage the use of language to ask for help in the early stages

Young children who have difficulty asking for help can be supported in the following ways:

💬 Create situations where the child needs to ask for help (eg getting dressed, opening a door, reaching a toy, taking a lid off a yoghurt pot or opening a container).

💬 Ask 'Do you want help?', supported with a Makaton sign (see Glossary) as appropriate.

💬 Encourage the child to imitate the word 'help' or the Makaton sign.

💬 Role play situations. For example, one adult sits with the child and another adult gives the child a task they won't be able to do themselves, such as taking the lid off a box. The adult sitting with the child signs and says 'Help' in order to model to the child how to ask for help.

💬 Emphasise both the word and the sign for 'help' when you are talking to other adults and children (eg 'Mary, can I have some *help* please?').

💬 Specifically praise the child when they spontaneously ask for help.

Speechmark

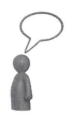

Expression

What do we mean by 'the functions of language'?

We use language for a variety of different functions – for example, to get a person's **attention**, to **greet** them, to **comment** on things happening around us, to **request** things that we want or to **say** 'no' to things we don't want. We can also ask for **help**. As we get older, we develop better and more appropriate ways to use language. However, children with social communication difficulties may find these skills difficult to learn. This can impact on the way they communicate with and respond to other people.

Children in the later stages of development who have difficulty using language for different functions may:

- struggle to get other people's attention appropriately

- not respond as expected when greeted and may be unsure of how to greet others

- have difficulty asking and answering questions effectively

- struggle to talk about events or activities: they can find it hard to process, plan and sequence language, which can mean that the listener may have difficulty following their narrative

- find it difficult to give the listener the right amount of information about an event (ie they give either too little or too much)

- have difficulty using language for more sophisticated purposes, such as humour, negotiation, explanation and reasoning.

- not know how to ask for clarification and help

- find it difficult to express their feelings and emotions.

Ways to encourage the use of language to ask for help in the later stages

💬 Explore with the child the range of situations in which people may need to ask for help (eg when they haven't understood, when something is too difficult, when they have made a mistake, when they are hurt or when they need emotional support).

💬 Talk about how it is OK to need help and that at some time everyone will.

💬 Discuss how people want to help and how they may feel upset if their offer of help is rejected in a rude manner.

💬 Discuss the ways in which different people show that they need help, and talk about which strategies work best.

💬 Try a range of strategies for asking for help to find one the child feels comfortable with (eg a card on the desk to turn over when they want some extra help, using a sign, putting up their hand).

💬 Use visual prompts (see Glossary) and Social Stories™ (Gray, 2001) to remind the child to use their strategies to ask for help.

All adults working with the child should know about the strategy the child is currently using to ask for help.

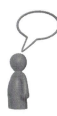

Expression

WORKSHEET 3

What do we mean by the disordered features of expressive language?

We use language for a variety of different functions: for example, to get a person's attention, to comment on things happening around us, to say 'no' or to request things and ask questions. As we get older, we learn the best and most appropriate ways to use language. Children with social communication difficulties may appear different from other children in the way they communicate with and respond to other people and in the range of functions of language they have. Some of their behaviours may mask difficulties with understanding spoken language. These difficulties can be subtle and therefore hard to identify. Although children with social communication difficulties may use a variety of words and sentences, they may not have a full understanding of the underlying meaning of what they are saying.

Children with disordered features of expressive language may present with some or all of the following:

- difficulties with using language for a range of functions (eg asking questions, seeking clarification, saying 'no', starting and ending a conversation)

- unusual language (eg they may produce 'adult-like' speech or precise sentences, or they may use 'made-up words' such as 'slicket')

- language produced from 'learned chunks' rather than used flexibly (ie they may memorise and over-use certain phrases)

- echolalia (ie they repeat what is said). This could either be immediate (they repeat what has been said straight after it has been said) or delayed (they may use a phrase from earlier on in the day)

- using repetitive language or asking a lot of questions, with little interest in the answers

- restricted interests that dominate conversations and play.

Speechmark

Ways to encourage a child to develop expressive language

- Provide opportunities for social play, both at home and at nursery or school.

- Highlight positive interactions between the child and their peers. Use specific praise (see Glossary) (eg 'That was good talking').

- Avoid asking the child to repeat phrases that you have said, as this reinforces echolalia or stereotypical language.

- Give the child opportunities to engage in pretend play, mime and role play (eg having a dolls' tea party). This supports development of creative language, flexibility, sequencing and narrative skills.

- Develop the child's awareness of others' interests and how these may not be the same as the child's own.

- During play, follow the child's lead rather than telling them what to do.

- Use clear and simple language relating to or describing what the child is playing with or doing in order to provide an appropriate language model.

- Reduce the number of questions that you ask the child; instead, comment on what they are doing.

- Don't reinforce 'made-up' words; instead, model the specific word for what is meant in the particular context.

- When offering choices (eg biscuit or banana), use objects or pictures as prompts.

- Give the child opportunities to practise language for various functions (eg for negotiation and for starting and ending conversations). Modelling these at different times during the day shows the child how flexible language can be.

Speechmark

Conversation Skills

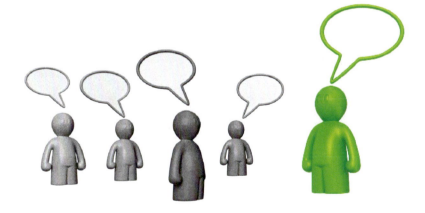

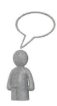

Verbal

HOW TO ENCOURAGE THE DEVELOPMENT OF CONVERSATION SKILLS – **STARTING A CONVERSATION**

4a

What are conversation skills and why are they important?

The ability to have conversations forms the basis of social interaction. Having conversations with one or more people involves a complex set of skills (both verbal and non-verbal). It develops from the early stages of turn taking between parent and infant and evolves into long and complex verbal conversations around a shared topic.

The skills involved in having conversations often require specific teaching in children with social communication difficulties.

Children who have difficulty with conversation skills may:

- have poor attention and listening skills

- have difficulty taking turns

- use inappropriate or unusual eye contact, body language or personal space

- find it difficult to talk on a range of subjects (particularly those that don't interest them) or may be unable to stay on topic (ie talk about the same thing as their conversation partner)

- have difficulty understanding and formulating questions

- have difficulty finding appropriate ways to start and finish conversations

- have difficulty joining conversations that are already taking place

- use few of the usual verbal and non-verbal behaviours to show that they are interested (eg nodding, using 'um' and 'uh-huh', asking questions and looking interested)

- be socially isolated and have difficulty making friends.

Ways to teach children how to start a conversation

The different skill areas can be taught individually to a child or as part of a small group activity. The generalisation and practice of all skills should be encouraged in as many different situations with as many different conversation partners as possible.

- Introduce games that encourage the use of greetings (eg pass a greeting from one person to another around a group, or ask the children to think of different ways to greet people).

- Introduce sorting between appropriate and inappropriate ways to start conversations (possible conversation openers could be written on to cards to be sorted).

- Use conversation cue cards (see Glossary) with suitable conversation starters written on them, such as 'Hello, how was your weekend?'

- Teach the meaning and use of 'wh-' questions (eg what, who, where, when) to start conversations.

- Practise different conversation starters through role play.

- Engineer situations in which a child has to approach others because you have created a need for that child to do so.

- Teach the non-verbal aspects of starting a conversation (eg where to stand, using a friendly face, using a friendly voice and making eye contact).

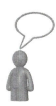

Verbal

WORKSHEET 4B

What are conversation skills and why are they important?

The ability to have conversations forms the basis of social interaction. Having conversations with one or more people involves a complex set of skills (both verbal and non-verbal). It develops from the early stages of turn taking between parent and infant and evolves into long and complex verbal conversations around a shared topic.

The skills involved in having conversations often require specific teaching in children with social communication difficulties.

Children who have difficulty with conversation skills may:

- have poor attention and listening skills

- have difficulty taking turns

- use inappropriate or unusual eye contact, body language or personal space

- find it difficult to talk on a range of subjects (particularly those that don't interest them) or may be unable to stay on topic (ie talk about the same thing as their conversation partner)

- have difficulty understanding and formulating questions

- have difficulty finding appropriate ways to start and finish conversations

- have difficulty joining conversations that are already taking place

- use few of the usual verbal and non-verbal behaviours to show that they are interested (eg nodding, using 'um' and 'uh-huh', asking questions and looking interested)

- be socially isolated and have difficulty making friends.

Ways to teach children how to join a conversation

The different skill areas can be taught individually to a child or as part of a small group activity. The generalisation and practice of all skills should be encouraged in as many different situations with as many different conversation partners as possible.

- Teach the 'rules' of joining in conversations (ie teach the child to watch, listen, move close, wait for a pause, talk about the same topic and maintain eye contact to show that they are interested).

- Use conversation cue cards (see Glossary) on which written and picture prompts remind the child of the 'rules'.

- Use a Social Stories™ (Gray, 2001) to teach about approaching another child to talk about their interest (eg ending with something like 'John will like it if I talk about football').

- Practise skills of joining in conversations through group games and role play.

- Use videos or DVDs to help the child to analyse how others join in conversations, and compare successful and unsuccesful ways of doing this.

- Create situations in which the child has to approach others because you have created a need for them to do so (eg to find out information or to pass on a message).

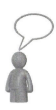

Verbal

WORKSHEET 4C

What are conversation skills and why are they important?

The ability to have conversations forms the basis of social interaction. Having conversations with one or more people involves a complex set of skills (both verbal and non-verbal). It develops from the early stages of turn taking between parent and infant and evolves into long and complex verbal conversations around a shared topic.

The skills involved in having conversations often require specific teaching in children with social communication difficulties.

Children who have difficulty with conversation skills may:

- have poor attention and listening skills

- have difficulty taking turns

- use inappropriate or unusual eye contact, body language or personal space

- find it difficult to talk on a range of subjects (particularly those that don't interest them) or may be unable to stay on topic (ie talk about the same thing as their conversation partner)

- have difficulty understanding and formulating questions

- have difficulty finding appropriate ways to start and finish conversations

- have difficulty joining conversations that are already taking place

- use few of the usual verbal and non-verbal behaviours to show they are interested (eg nodding, using 'um' and 'uh-huh', asking questions and looking interested)

- be socially isolated and have difficulty making friends.

Ways to teach children how to keep a conversation going

The different skill areas can be taught individually to a child or as part of a small group activity. The generalisation and practice of all skills should be encouraged in as many different situations with as many different conversation partners as possible.

- Use circle time games (see Glossary) to promote listening and responding to others.

- Use role play to demonstrate the importance of non-verbal signals that indicate interest (eg nodding, saying 'uh-huh' and looking at the person who is talking).

- Practise asking questions on a given topic, such as personal interests and weekend news.

- Use circle time games or role play to practise taking turns in a conversation.

- Use *Comic Strip Conversations* (Gray, 1994) to illustrate the need for the child to be thinking and talking about the same thing as their conversational partner, and to show turn taking and keeping to the topic.

- Teach strategies individually and through role play to repair conversations when breakdown has occurred due to misunderstanding, disagreement or assumed knowledge. Help the child to identify what went wrong (where the misunderstanding was) and how they can 'mend' it.

Speechmark

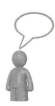

Verbal

HOW TO ENCOURAGE THE DEVELOPMENT OF CONVERSATION SKILLS – **ENDING A CONVERSATION**

4d

What are conversation skills and why are they important?

The ability to have conversations forms the basis of social interaction. Having conversations with one or more people involves a complex set of skills (both verbal and non-verbal). It develops from the early stages of turn taking between parent and infant and evolves into long and complex verbal conversations around a shared topic.

The skills involved in having conversations often require specific teaching in children with social communication difficulties.

Children who have difficulty with conversation skills may:

- have poor attention and listening skills

- have difficulty taking turns

- use inappropriate or unusual eye contact, body language or personal space

- find it difficult to talk on a range of subjects (particularly those that don't interest them) or may be unable to stay on topic (ie talk about the same thing as their conversation partner)

- have difficulty understanding and formulating questions

- have difficulty finding appropriate ways to start and finish conversations

- have difficulty joining conversations that are already taking place

- use few of the usual verbal and non-verbal behaviours to show they are interested (eg nodding, using 'um' and 'uh-huh', asking questions and looking interested)

- be socially isolated and have difficulty making friends.

45

WORKSHEET 4D

Ways to teach children how to end a conversation

The different skill areas can be taught individually to a child or as part of a small group activity. The generalisation and practice of all skills should be encouraged in as many different situations with as many different conversation partners as possible.

- Teach the child (through role play) how to read the non-verbal signs that the listener wants to end the conversation (eg looking away, moving away, checking their watch).

- In a small group, adults demonstrate (through role play) poor skills at ending conversations (eg walking away without saying anything, looking bored and not talking). Ask for suggestions from the group and have the children practise using appropriate or better skills in pairs.

- Create situations (either through role play or in everyday situations) in which the adult continues to try to have a conversation even when it is clear that the child wants to do something else, and then model the appropriate way to end the conversation.

- Show DVDs or videos that demonstrate different ways in which conversations are ended and, as a group, rate these ways according to their effectiveness.

- Use specific praise (see Glossary) to draw attention to appropriate ways to end conversations.

- Teach key phrases and use conversation cue cards (see Glossary) as reminders.

Speechmark

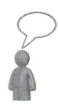

Verbal

HOW TO ENCOURAGE THE DEVELOPMENT OF CONVERSATION SKILLS – **REPAIRING A CONVERSATION** WHEN THINGS GO WRONG

4e

What are conversation skills and why are they important?

The ability to have conversations forms the basis of social interaction. Having conversations with one or more people involves a complex set of skills (both verbal and non-verbal). It develops from the early stages of turn taking between parent and infant and evolves into long and complex verbal conversations around a shared topic.

The skills involved in having conversations often require specific teaching in children with social communication difficulties.

Children who have difficulty with conversation skills may:

- have poor attention and listening skills

- have difficulty taking turns

- use inappropriate or unusual eye contact, body language or personal space

- find it difficult to talk on a range of subjects (particularly those that don't interest them) or may be unable to stay on topic (ie talk about the same thing as their conversation partner)

- have difficulty understanding and formulating questions

- have difficulty finding appropriate ways to start and finish conversations

- have difficulty joining conversations that are already taking place

- use few of the usual verbal and non-verbal behaviours to show that they are interested (eg nodding, using 'um' and 'uh-huh', asking questions and looking interested)

- be socially isolated and have difficulty making friends.

Ways to teach children how to repair conversations

For conversations to be successful, both conversation partners have to recognise when a misunderstanding occurs and how to address it. This skill is known as 'repair' and may need to be specifically taught to children with social communication difficulties.

- Explain that all conversations can break down at some point – give examples using video, television programmes or role play, or point out real-life examples as they occur.

- To prevent misunderstanding, it is important that the child gives all the contextual information that the listener needs (see Handout 9a 'How to develop an understanding of listener needs').

- Through role play and pictures of people in emotional situations, teach the body language, facial expressions and intonation of voice that indicate that someone is confused, so that the child is able to recognise this in another person.

- Use a visual prompt or cue card (see Glossary) to prompt the child to say when they haven't understood a word or phrase. Within separate activities, present novel or difficult words as opportunities to encourage this skill.

- Teach about and practise questions that can be asked to gain more information on a subject. Initially, this could be done through games such as 'Give Us a Clue' (see Glossary) and then practised within conversations (see Handout 2h 'How to encourage the development of the functions of language – questioning').

- Teach set phrases, such as 'Do you understand?' or 'You look confused'.

- Teach strategies for clarifying information (eg asking the speaker to talk more slowly, give more contextual information, rephrase or repeat certain points).

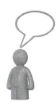

Non-verbal

Why is eye contact important?

- It helps direct attention.

- It shows others that you are listening.

- It helps regulate conversation.

- It is necessary for picking up non-verbal information, such as facial expression.

Children with social communication difficulties often find it difficult to look and listen at the same time, and report that it can be very stressful for them. So, while eye contact should be encouraged as a social skill, it should NOT BE ENFORCED. It may be helpful to teach a strategy of looking near a person's eyes rather than directly into them. Although it may be difficult for some children, they do need to understand the importance of eye contact in social situations. It is helpful if everyone knows that eye contact is stressful for the child and that they are not being stubborn or rude.

Children who have difficulty with eye contact may:

- not make eye contact when expected

- make unusual use of eye contact (eg over-use and staring as well as reduced eye contact)

- actively avoid eye contact by turning away.

Be aware that just because a child is not looking at you, this does not mean that they are not listening or are not interested. Check that the child is listening by asking questions.

Ways to encourage eye contact in the early stages

Activities should be simple and motivating for the child. Remember not to enforce eye contact, but just to encourage it.

- When playing a motivating game (eg bubble blowing), wait for the child to look towards you before you respond.

- Use repeated phrases or words to encourage the child to look at you (eg 'Ready …').

- Bring the toy or object up to your eye level to encourage the child to look at you.

- Use attention-grabbing toys and objects (eg sparkly, noisy or fast-moving toys).

- Play 'Peek-a-Boo' games.

- Sing action songs (eg 'Row Your Boat') and stop and wait for the child to look at you before continuing.

- Play tickling or bouncing games, which need eye contact to keep them going.

- Look in a mirror together – some children are more comfortable making eye contact via a mirror rather than face to face.

Speechmark

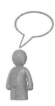

Non-verbal

5b

WORKSHEET 5B

Why is eye contact important?

- It helps direct attention.

- It shows others that you are listening.

- It helps regulate conversation.

- It is necessary for picking up non-verbal information, such as facial expression.

Children with social communication difficulties often find it difficult to look and listen at the same time, and report that it can be very stressful for them. So, while eye contact should be encouraged as a social skill, it should NOT BE ENFORCED. It may be helpful to teach a strategy of looking near a person's eyes rather than directly into them. Although it may be difficult for some children, they do need to understand the importance of eye contact in social situations. It is helpful if everyone knows that eye contact is stressful for the child and that they are not being stubborn or rude.

Children who have difficulty with eye contact may:

- not make eye contact when expected

- make unusual use of eye contact (eg over-use and staring as well as reduced eye contact)

- actively avoid eye contact by turning away.

Be aware that just because a child is not looking at you, this does not mean that they are not listening or are not interested. Check that the child is listening by asking questions.

Ways to encourage eye contact in the intermediate stage

Activities should be simple and motivating for the child. Remember not to enforce eye contact, but just to encourage it.

- Be specific about the language used to encourage eye contact (eg 'Look at the person who's talking' rather than 'Look at the teacher').

- Use specific praise (see Glossary) (eg 'Good looking') or verbal prompts, as well as visual prompts (see Glossary) (eg signs or symbols).

- Play group games, such as 'When I Look at You ...', 'Eye Swap Chairs' and 'Pass the Blink' (from *The Social Use of Language Programme*: Rinaldi, 1995).

- Play games such as 'Simon Says' and miming or copying games (arrange the children in pairs, with one child doing the actions and the other being the mirror).

- Organise role play games and dressing up.

- Look in a mirror together – some children are more comfortable making eye contact via a mirror rather than face to face.

- Use 'sabotage' (see Glossary) or delayed response (ie delay offering an item until eye contact is made).

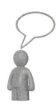

Non-verbal

Why is eye contact important?

- It helps direct attention.

- It shows others that you are listening.

- It helps regulate conversation.

- It is necessary for picking up non-verbal information, such as facial expression.

Children with social communication difficulties often find it difficult to look and listen at the same time, and report that it can be very stressful for them. So, while eye contact should be encouraged as a social skill, it should NOT BE ENFORCED. It may be helpful to teach a strategy of looking near a person's eyes rather than directly into them. Although it may be difficult for some children, they do need to understand the importance of eye contact in social situations. It is helpful if everyone knows that eye contact is stressful for the child and that they are not being stubborn or rude.

Children who have difficulty with eye contact may:

- not make eye contact when expected

- make unusual use of eye contact (eg over-use and staring as well as reduced eye contact)

- actively avoid eye contact by turning away.

Be aware that just because a child is not looking at you, this does not mean that they are not listening or are not interested. Check that the child is listening by asking questions.

Ways to encourage eye contact in the later stages

Remember not to enforce eye contact, but just to encourage it. Use specific praise (see Glossary) (eg 'Good looking') and gestures or signs to encourage use of eye contact. Consider group eye contact games (see Glossary), which emphasise looking. At this stage, it is helpful to give children the reasons why eye contact is important.

- Model appropriate eye contact through role play or video and how things can go wrong if appropriate eye contact is not made.

- Use role play and drama so that the child can practise appropriate use of eye contact.

- Agree coping strategies with the child (eg to look at eyebrows if looking directly into eyes is uncomfortable).

- Teach the child to tell people if they have difficulty looking and listening at the same time. Consider including this in a communication passport (see Glossary).

- Play games to practise using eye contact, such as 'Wink Murder', 'Changeabout', 'Pass the Facial Expression', 'Eye Swap Chairs' and '1-2-3 Look!' (from *The Social Use of Language Programme*: Rinaldi, 1995).

- Make use of visual cue cards and conversation cue cards (see Glossary).

- Use repetitive phrases (eg '1-2-3 Look at me') that remind the child about making eye contact in group situations.

Speechmark

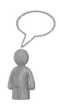

Non-verbal

What are turn-taking skills and why are they important?

Turn-taking skills are the basis of social interaction between two or more people. Turn-taking skills develop in infancy when a young baby listens to its parent and then attempts to copy lip and tongue movements and vocalisations.

Turn-taking skills develop in play as well as in interaction. A child will learn to take turns with a toy, when speaking with an adult and then in conversations with peers.

Many young children find it difficult to learn to wait, share and take turns. These skills are used throughout a person's life as a social skill (ie what is acceptable behaviour in society) and to aid effective communication (conversations soon break down if two people keep on talking at the same time).

Children with delayed development of turn-taking skills:

- have difficulty sharing toys, activities and someone's attention

- may find it difficult to work as part of a group, particularly if this involves waiting for their turn

- may call out answers and take longer than usual to learn to put up their hand in school

- have difficulty managing social interaction, particularly conversations.

Ways to encourage turn-taking skills in the early stages

Activities should be simple and motivating for the child. Remember to leave time for the child to respond before prompting them. Use the language of turn taking (eg 'Your turn', 'Mummy's turn'), with the appropriate sign, gesture or visual prompt or cue card (see Glossary). Build up gradually from working one-to-one to working in small groups. Start with very simple activities, introducing more complex ones as you progress. For example, with the child:

- build a tower, taking turns to add bricks

- roll a car or ball between you

- take turns to press the button on cause–effect toys (eg musical toys, spinning tops, pop-up toys)

- take turns with puzzle pieces

- take turns playing musical instruments

- take turns using colours to make a picture or pattern

- imitate actions (eg clapping, waving, jumping) with or without a mirror

- have pretend conversations on a telephone

- copy sounds (eg babble, animal noises and other symbolic noises, singing).

Speechmark

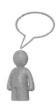

Non-verbal

WORKSHEET 5E

What are turn-taking skills and why are they important?

Turn-taking skills are the basis of social interaction between two or more people. Turn-taking skills develop in infancy when a young baby listens to its parent and then attempts to copy lip and tongue movements and vocalisations.

Turn-taking skills develop in play as well as in interaction. A child will learn to take turns with a toy, when speaking with an adult and then in conversations with peers.

Many young children find it difficult to learn to wait, share and take turns. These skills are used throughout a person's life as a social skill (ie what is acceptable behaviour in society) and to aid effective communication (conversations soon break down if two people keep on talking at the same time).

Children with delayed development of turn-taking skills:

- have difficulty sharing toys, activities and someone's attention

- may find it difficult to work as part of a group, particularly if this involves waiting for their turn

- may call out answers and take longer than usual to learn to put up their hand in school

- have difficulty managing social interaction, particularly conversations.

Ways to encourage turn-taking skills in groups

Once children have achieved turn taking on a one-to-one basis, encourage generalisation of these skills to working with other children and small groups. It is important to use the language of turn taking (eg 'Whose turn is it now?', 'It's Matthew's turn'). Use visual support, such as gesture and symbols (eg pointing to individual children as they take their turns, using a 'wait' card and a 'hand up' card to prompt). Children should be motivated to want a turn, and time between turns should not be too long initially.

💬 Many of the simple turn-taking activities, such as ball rolling, passing an object, playing a musical instrument, lifting a flap in a story book, putting a brick on a tower, taking a turn in a fishing game and playing a posting game, can be applied to group situations.

💬 Encourage a child to listen for their name in a group (eg for their turn to pop bubbles).

💬 Tell or show children where to sit. Some children find sitting in a group easier if they know where to sit (eg a cushion, carpet square or specific chair).

💬 Sing action songs in which children take turns at choosing the action (eg 'Here We Go Round the Mulberry Bush', 'Old Macdonald Had a Farm').

💬 Take turns to say parts of a familiar nursery rhyme or to tell a familiar story, making sure each child has a turn at saying something (ie the activity is shared around the group).

Speechmark

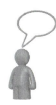

Non-verbal

WORKSHEET 5F

What are turn-taking skills and why are they important?

Turn-taking skills are the basis of social interaction between two or more people. Turn-taking skills develop in infancy when a young baby listens to its parent and then attempts to copy lip and tongue movements and vocalisations.

Turn-taking skills develop in play as well as in interaction. A child will learn to take turns with a toy, when speaking with an adult and then in conversations with peers.

Many young children find it difficult to learn to wait, share and take turns. These skills are used throughout a person's life as a social skill (ie what is acceptable behaviour in society) and to aid effective communication (conversations soon break down if two people keep on talking at the same time).

Children with delayed development of turn-taking skills:

- have difficulty sharing toys, activities and someone's attention

- may find it difficult to work as part of a group, particularly if this involves waiting for their turn

- may call out answers and take longer than usual to learn to put up their hand in school

- have difficulty managing social interaction, particularly conversations.

Ways to encourage turn-taking skills in conversations

Some children have difficulty taking turns in conversations; they may like to talk at length about subjects that interest them, not know how to keep a conversation going or have difficulty joining conversations. These children may need to be specifically taught the rules of conversation individually or in small groups. These skills can be taught through games and role play. Conversation cue cards (see Glossary) can support generalisation of these skills. The following is a list of some of the important rules to teach:

- Look at the person who is speaking and show that you are interested by nodding, saying 'Really?' or 'Mm' and asking questions. Using a friendly face will also show them that you are interested.

- Look at the person while you speak – nod and agree with the speaker and then wait for a pause.

- Talk about the same thing as the other person.

- Don't talk for too long – stop after you've made one or two points.

- Give the other person a chance to respond to what you are saying.

Speechmark

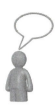

Non-verbal

HOW TO ENCOURAGE THE UNDERSTANDING AND USE OF **FACIAL EXPRESSION**

5g

Why is it important to understand and be able to use appropriate facial expressions?

We communicate a great deal using facial expression. We can convey a wide range of feelings, such as sadness, happiness, anxiety and disbelief, using just our faces. We support our own verbal communication with expressions and also interpret the moods and intentions of others from the facial expressions they use when speaking to us.

When used appropriately, facial expressions match spoken communication as well as other forms of non-verbal communication, such as gesture and body language.

Children who have difficulty understanding and using facial expressions may:

- appear to have a blank ('deadpan') expression of disinterest

- have difficulty matching their facial expression to their verbal expression (eg smiling while saying something sad)

- use facial expressions that are inappropriate to the situation, such as looking happy when being told off

- misinterpret other people's facial expressions and therefore misunderstand situations.

Ways to help the understanding and use of facial expressions

Children who have these difficulties need to be specifically taught how to use and recognise each separate expression.

- Use photos or pictures to identify different facial expressions. Begin with real-life photos or pictures – sort them into categories of emotions to reinforce the vocabulary of emotions and feelings.

- Talk about what each part of the face does during different expressions (eg 'angry eyebrows', 'smiling mouth', 'sad eyes').

- Use an 'Identikit' face (www.do2learn.com) to piece together different facial expressions to match different emotions.

- Use drama and role play to show how different expressions are relevant to different situations.

- Play games such as 'Pass the Expression' (see Glossary), in which a group take it in turns to copy each other's facial expressions.

- Use video and/or books and talk about characters' facial expressions, relating them to the situations in the story and why they feel the way they do.

- Use mirror work to help children become more aware of their own facial expressions.

- Label emotions as a child experiences them to help the child associate the vocabulary with the feeling.

Non-verbal

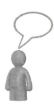

HOW TO ENCOURAGE THE UNDERSTANDING AND USE OF **BODY LANGUAGE**

5h

Why is it important to understand and use appropriate body language?

When we communicate with others we use a great deal of non-verbal communication, such as facial expression and body language. Subtle changes in a person's stance or movements can indicate changes in the meaning of what is being said or the emotions a person is experiencing. For example, a person speaking with their hands on their hips may be angry, a person who asks a question and spreads their arms wide is inviting answers, and someone with their head resting on their hands might be bored.

Children who struggle with aspects of social communication may find it difficult to interpret the body movements and gestures of other people, as well as to use their own body language appropriately.

Children who have difficulty using and interpreting body language may:

- not associate a person's body movements with what they are saying

- not understand the intention of what is being said as they interpret the words literally and don't pick up on cues of body language (eg they may not understand what it means if the speaker also has their arms folded)

- under-use or over-use their own body movements

- not be aware of how body language and gesture can support or reinforce what is being said

- not recognise the feelings of others because they are unable to interpret their body language (eg they may not understand that hands over the face may mean that a person is upset or that turning or looking away may mean that a person doesn't want to talk)

- not always be aware of personal space (eg they may stand too close).

WORKSHEET 5H

Ways to encourage the understanding and use of body language

Children with difficulties in this area may need to be specifically taught what different postures and movements mean.

- Identify postures and movements as a person makes them and discuss what they may mean. Include conventional gestures, such as nodding and shaking the head and beckoning.

- Use a mirror to help the child to recognise body language and to practise relevant movements.

- Look at photos and discuss how we know what a person is feeling without needing to hear what they are saying.

- Practise saying different things with the right body language (eg 'I am very excited').

- Encourage the child to look at people during the day and to make 'guesses' about how those people are feeling, based on what the child can see.

- Use mime, role play and drama to practise different postures and movements and demonstrate personal boundaries.

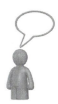

Non-verbal

HOW TO DEVELOP AWARENESS OF **PERSONAL SPACE** (PROXIMITY)

5i

Why is it important to understand and be able to respect personal space?

In order to interact successfully with others we need to be able to recognise, understand and respect our own and other people's personal space. This involves positioning ourselves at appropriate distances from others when interacting. It also involves gestures, such as appropriate hugging and touching. Different distances are appropriate for different situations and for different relationships (eg you may have to stand closer than usual to a stranger if you are in a crowded place or sit closer to a parent than you would to a teacher).

Children who have difficulty understanding and respecting their own and other people's personal space may:

- sit or stand too close, causing the listener to feel uncomfortable, which could create a negative impression

- stand too far away and therefore the listener may not be aware of the child's attempt to communicate with them

- use inappropriate touching and hugging etc, which could cause the other person to feel uncomfortable

- become distressed if other people come too close to them or touch them.

Ways to help children understand their own and other people's personal space

Children with these difficulties may need to be specifically taught the rules of personal space. They may need to be taught individually at first and then through small group work.

- Explain how others can feel when someone stands too close.

- Demonstrate appropriate and inappropriate personal space (eg using puppets, soft toys and miniatures).

- Identify appropriate and inappropriate personal space through circle time activities (see Glossary) (eg passing messages).

- Write a Social Story™ (Gray, 2001) for the child, explaining why it is important to stand at the right distance from someone when talking to them.

- Practise using appropriate personal space during role play, drama, music, movement, miming or similar activities.

- Watch television dramas, videos and films, for example, and discuss the use of personal space between characters.

- Look at pictures in magazines and books and, again, discuss the use of personal space between people in the pictures.

- Use prompts and reminders in general conversation if appropriate.

- Teach the child to read other people's non-verbal signs of discomfort.

- Teach the child to say when they are uncomfortable with someone being too close – teaching a set phrase might be helpful (eg 'It makes me uncomfortable when people get too close to me').

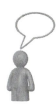

Non-verbal

Why is it important to understand and use appropriate intonation patterns during conversation?

By using specific intonation when we talk, we can convey different meanings and emotions. For example, a rising intonation at the end of a sentence can imply a question, and sarcasm is often conveyed through intonation. By changing the 'tone' of an utterance, we change the meaning of the actual words. We need to be able to interpret intonation in order to be able to understand all elements of spoken language, and we need to be able to use intonation in order to accurately convey a full range of meanings and emotions.

Children who have difficulty understanding and using intonation may:

- have a monotone voice (i.e. the voice sounds flat), which can make them difficult to listen to as well as making them sound uninterested

- be misinterpreted because their tone doesn't match what they are saying

- misread situations by not understanding the tone of the speaker

- become isolated because other children find it difficult to remain focused on what they are saying.

Ways to help the understanding and use of intonation

Children who have difficulty understanding and using intonation will need to be specifically taught how to interpret and use it in their own speech.

- Use drama and role play to demonstrate a range of intonation patterns.

- Use pictures of facial expressions to match to tone of voice.

- Use audio and video resources to listen to and identify various tones.

- Read books out loud using exaggerated tones for characters' speech.

- Use puppets (eg Punch and Judy) to act out simple scenarios with relevant intonation.

- Practise changing voice pitch, moving from high to low pitch and back again.

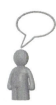

Non-verbal

Why is gesture important?

Gestures are body movements, often made with the hand or arm, which are used both with and without speech to convey messages (eg waving to mean 'Bye' and beckoning to mean 'Come over here'). An accompanying facial expression often completes the meaning. Gestures are a crucial part of everyday communication, such as chatting, giving directions, giving instructions and describing events. Gestures are culture specific and can vary between societies and social groups.

Children who have difficulty with gesture:

- often don't use early gestures, such as pointing or holding their arms up to be lifted, when younger

- don't recognise or understand what others are saying through their gestures

- may seem unusual or unnatural because they don't use gestures at all or they use them at inappropriate times or with the wrong person

- may use odd or over-exaggerated gestures

- may use inappropriate gestures that do not match the content of what they are saying or are unsuitable in the current context

- may miss non-verbal information given through gestures during conversation

- may become confused by gestures that are not explicit.

WORKSHEET 5K

Ways to encourage the use of gestures in the early stages

- Teach a child to point and follow another's pointing.

- Use gestures as well as words and wait for a response (eg ask 'Do you want to come up?', while holding your arms out; then pause and, still holding your arms out, ask 'Coming up?').

- Use the same gesture repeatedly in regular situations (eg place your index finger on your palm before playing 'Round and Round the Garden'; show the 'all gone' gesture when food is finished).

- Wait for the child to use a whole body movement to ask for something to be repeated (eg a bouncing game).

- Model gestures for songs and rhymes (eg a circular movement for 'The Wheels on the Bus').

- Use gestures when talking (eg point to Daddy as you say 'Daddy').

- Sing rhymes and songs and accompany these with actions, encouraging the child to join in.

- Model the gesture for 'Come here' rather than pulling the child by the hand.

- A formal signing system such as Makaton (see Glossary) may be useful.

70

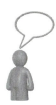

Non-verbal

HOW TO ENCOURAGE THE USE OF **GESTURE** – LATER STAGES

5l

Why is gesture important?

Gestures are body movements, often made with the hand or arm, which are used both with and without speech to convey messages (eg waving to mean 'Bye' and beckoning to mean 'Come over here'). An accompanying facial expression often completes the meaning. Gestures are a crucial part of everyday communication, such as chatting, giving directions, giving instructions and describing events. Gestures are culture specific and can vary between societies and social groups.

Children who have difficulty with gesture:

- often don't use early gestures, such as pointing or holding their arms up to be lifted, when younger

- don't recognise or understand what others are saying through their gestures

- may seem unusual or unnatural because they don't use gestures at all or they use them at inappropriate times or with the wrong person

- may use odd or over-exaggerated gestures

- may use inappropriate gestures that don't match the content of what they are saying or are unsuitable in the current context

- may miss non-verbal information given through gestures during conversation

- may become confused by gestures that are not explicit.

Ways to encourage the use of gestures in the later stages

- Teach age-appropriate gestures so that the child, is not excluded from this form of communication, and make these gestures easy to copy (eg 'High Five' – use the child's peers for reference).

- Tell the child when to use gestures.

- Role play to practise gestures and the words that may be used with them.

- Prompt the child to use gestures in real-life situations.

- Prompt the child to use gestures in different situations (eg to greet a friend, to get someone's attention or say goodbye).

- Help the child to develop their understanding of the gestures used by others.

Speechmark

Social Skills

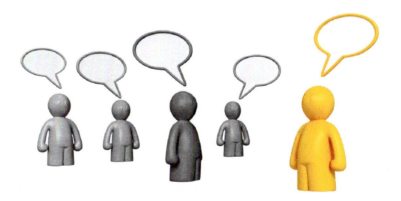

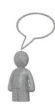

Social interaction

WORKSHEET 6A

Why is it important to understand and be able to express emotions?

In order to interact successfully with others we need to be able to recognise and understand a range of emotions, both in ourselves and in other people, as well as be able to express emotions. Emotions can be understood and expressed verbally and non-verbally (eg through tone of voice, facial expression and body language).

These skills develop as children mature. While younger children will understand and express basic emotions (happy, sad), older children will understand and express a wider range of more complex emotions (amusement, frustration).

Children who have difficulty understanding and expressing emotions may:

- have difficulty understanding and expressing their own emotions, which can lead to difficulties in recognising and understanding these emotions in those around them

- appear detached or unaware even when others are hurt, may laugh inappropriately and do things that appear rude or hurtful

- struggle to understand and use body language appropriately

- struggle to understand and use facial expression appropriately

- have difficulty distinguishing one emotion from another (eg telling the difference between upset and cross)

- have difficulty controlling their emotions (eg angry outbursts).

Speechmark

Ways to help the understanding of basic emotions

At a young age, children can show emotions such as enjoyment, fear and anger. They are able to interpret some emotional expressions in familiar adults. As they mature, they develop understanding and expression of obvious humour (eg slapstick). They are able to interpret emotions from facial expression and intonation.

- Name emotions as they are experienced in the child and others (eg 'You are a happy boy', 'Mummy's cross').

- Talk about the emotions of characters in books and photos and on television.

- Use photos and simple drawings to identify emotions (eg happy face, sad face).

- Use a mirror to practise recognising and making simple facial expressions.

- Adapt songs to highlight physical responses to emotions (eg 'If you're happy and you know it clap your hands, if you're angry and you know it stamp your feet').

- Use puppets to practise recognising and understanding emotions and feelings.

- Use 'time out' spaces or individual workstations for children who are prone to outbursts, to help them avoid emotional overload.

Speechmark

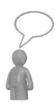

Social interaction

WORKSHEET 6B

Why is it important to understand and be able to express emotions?

In order to interact successfully with others we need to be able to recognise and understand a range of emotions, both in ourselves and in other people, as well as be able to express emotions. Emotions can be understood and expressed verbally and non-verbally (eg through tone of voice, facial expression and body language).

These skills develop as children mature. While younger children will understand and express basic emotions (happy, sad), older children will understand and express a wider range of more complex emotions (amusement, frustration).

Children who have difficulty understanding and expressing emotions may:

- have difficulty understanding and expressing their own emotions, which can lead to difficulties in recognising and understanding these emotions in those around them

- appear detached or unaware even when others are hurt, may laugh inappropriately and do things that appear rude or hurtful

- struggle to understand and use body language appropriately

- struggle to understand and use facial expression appropriately

- have difficulty distinguishing one emotion from another (eg telling the difference between upset and cross)

- have difficulty controlling their emotions (eg angry outbursts).

Ways to help the understanding of more complex emotions

Once children have an understanding of basic emotions, this develops into the ability to understand and express a wide range of more complex emotions (eg envy and embarrassment). Children who have difficulty recognising and understanding emotions may have particular difficulty in group situations. At this level, recognition of different emotional states can be very difficult as the differences can be expressed in a very subtle manner.

- Talk about emotions (possibly in small groups) – name and describe them and their effects on the body (eg tension, blushing), using pictures that illustrate different emotions.

- Role play different emotions, paying particular attention to facial expression, body posture and tone of voice (this can also be done through drama).

- Use *Comic Strip Conversations* (Gray, 1994) to speculate on how others might feel, and why.

- Use visual support (pictures on an emotions wheel or chart) to help identify current feelings. This can be extended to helping predict feelings in different or impending situations (eg exams). Emotions can be colour coded according to whether they are 'comfortable' or 'uncomfortable'.

- Use a Social Story™ (Gray, 2001) to teach a desired response to a specific situation (eg feeling calm in the playground).

- Use 'time out' spaces or individual workstations for children who are prone to outbursts, to help them avoid emotional overload.

- Use computer programs that can allow a child to change different aspects of facial expression (eyes, mouth, angle of head, etc), such as that found on www.do2learn.com.

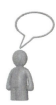

Social interaction

WORKSHEET 6C

How does play typically develop and why is it important?

Development of play skills is vital as this is how children learn about themselves, each other and the world. Play usually develops following a typical pattern, with early play being exploratory (touching and mouthing toys) and cause-and-effect (realising that an action has a consequence, such as pushing a button to make a toy pop up). Children then develop relational play (putting objects together, such as a spoon in a cup or teddy in a box) and begin to relate toys to both themselves and each other (eg giving teddy a drink). Play is then extended into sequential play (feeding dolly then putting her to bed) and symbolic play, in which one object represents another. Finally, imaginary and make-believe play develops.

As play develops, a child moves from playing by themselves to playing alongside others and, finally, interactively with other children, which is when many social skills develop, such as sharing, taking turns and listening to each other.

Children who have difficulty interacting may:

- appear isolated in the classroom and playground

- demonstrate play typical of younger children (eg cause-and-effect play) and are therefore not developmentally ready to engage in social and interactive play

- have difficulties sharing toys and may grab toys from other children

- prefer to play by themselves or with an adult

- have difficulties joining in with games appropriately, and therefore appear as withdrawn or aggressive.

Ways to develop interactive play skills in the early stages

💬 Ensure that there are opportunities for the child to take part in free play as well as structured play sessions.

💬 Put aside time (5–10 minutes) when you and the child play together; copy what the child is doing, using appropriate, simple language to comment on what they are doing.

💬 Join in with the child's play and model additional ideas in order to extend their play.

💬 During a play session you could comment on another child's play in order to stimulate interest in what another child is doing.

💬 In small groups play turn-taking games, praising the child when they wait for their turn, share toys, etc.

💬 Ensure that you use specific praise (see Glossary) when you see the child doing something well (eg 'good sharing', 'good talking').

💬 Ensure that the child has opportunities to observe other children playing appropriately.

💬 Encourage home corner play where roles are taken on (eg making telephone calls, taking an order for food).

💬 Use identical sets of equipment to model play sequences for the child to copy ('Identiplay', Phillips and Beavan, 2007).

Speechmark Ⓢ

Social interaction

HOW TO ENCOURAGE THE DEVELOPMENT OF
INTERACTIVE PLAY – LATER STAGES

6d

How does play typically develop and why is it important?

Development of play skills is vital as this is how children learn about themselves, each other and the world. Play usually develops following a typical pattern, with early play being exploratory (touching and mouthing toys) and cause-and-effect (realising that an action has a consequence, such as pushing a button to make a toy pop up). Children then develop relational play (putting objects together, such as a spoon in a cup or teddy in a box) and begin to relate toys to both themselves and each other (eg giving teddy a drink). Play is then extended into sequential play (feeding dolly, then putting her to bed) and symbolic play, in which one object represents another. Finally, imaginary and make-believe play develops.

As play develops, a child moves from playing by themselves to playing alongside others and, finally, interactively with other children, which is when many social skills develop (such as sharing, taking turns and listening to each other).

From age three upwards, children will typically start to engage in pretend play (eg doctors and nurses) with a group of other children; they may become involved in organising and cooperating during play and will also take part in games that have rules, and will follow these rules.

Children who have difficulty interacting may:

- appear isolated in the classroom and playground

- demonstrate play typical of younger children (eg cause-and-effect play) and are therefore not developmentally ready to engage in social- and interactive-type play

- have difficulties sharing toys and games and may grab toys from other children

- prefer to play by themselves or with an adult

- have difficulties with joining in with games appropriately, and therefore appear as withdrawn or aggressive.

Ways to develop interactive play skills in the later stages

💬 Create opportunities in the playground for children to become involved in structured games, which could be led by an adult.

💬 Join in with the child's play and model additional ideas in order to extend their play.

💬 During a play session you could comment on another child's play in order to stimulate interest in what another child is doing.

💬 Pair children up with a suitable role model who can support their interaction skills.

💬 In small groups play turn-taking games, praising the child when they wait for their turn, share toys, etc.

💬 Ensure that you use specific praise (see Glossary) when you see the child doing something well (eg 'good sharing', 'good talking').

💬 Ensure that the child has opportunities to observe other children playing and interacting appropriately – use peer praise (praising other children in the group) to highlight the behaviours you would like to see, for example praising another child in the group for demonstrating 'good sharing'.

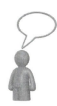

Social interaction

HOW TO ENCOURAGE THE DEVELOPMENT OF **SHARING** – EARLY STAGES

6e

What is sharing and why is it difficult for some children?

Sharing is a difficult concept for young children to learn. It is a skill that requires empathy (the ability to see things from another's perspective) and the ability to take turns and understand consequences and social expectations. Most children will need support at one time or another to be able to share toys and games; however, children with social communication difficulties need much more support and to be explicitly taught rules and boundaries.

Children who have difficulty sharing may:

- demonstrate play typical of younger children and are therefore not developmentally ready to engage in social- and interactive-type play

- be possessive about favourite toys and become distressed if other children have them

- grab toys from other children

- observe other children playing with the toy they want, but do not have strategies to ask for a turn

- prefer to play by themselves or with an adult

- have difficulties with joining in with games appropriately, and therefore appear as withdrawn or aggressive.

WORKSHEET 6E

Ways to encourage sharing in the early stages

- It is often easier for children to start being able to share with another adult. Therefore have one-to-one sessions with the child and gradually introduce another child into a session.

- Ensure that you use specific and immediate praise (see Glossary) when you see the child doing 'good sharing' (eg 'Well done, John, I like the way you let Robert have a go at playing with the car – good sharing').

- During a play session you could comment on other children's ability to share equipment and toys successfully.

- Consider using a visual cue (eg a sand timer) to support the child to play for a limited time with a toy, which is then passed on to another child.

- In small groups play turn-taking games, praising the child when they wait for their turn and pass a toy on.

- When doing activities such as painting, make sure there is enough equipment to go round!

- Try putting children in pairs and giving them one activity (eg a puzzle) between them. Support them to take turns – this will help them to understand the advantages of reaching a common goal together.

- Ensure that the child has opportunities to observe other children sharing appropriately – use peer praise (praising other children in the group) to highlight the behaviours you would like to see.

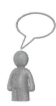

Social interaction

HOW TO ENCOURAGE THE DEVELOPMENT OF **SHARING** – LATER STAGES

6f

What skills do we need in order to 'share'?

Sharing is a difficult concept for young children to learn. It is a skill that requires empathy (the ability to see things from another's perspective) and the ability to take turns and understand consequences and social expectations. Most children will need support at one time or another to be able to share toys and games; however' children with social communication difficulties need much more support and need to be explicitly taught rules and boundaries.

Children who have difficulty sharing may:

- demonstrate play typical of younger children and are therefore not developmentally ready to engage in social- and interactive-type play

- be possessive about favourite toys and become distressed if other children have them

- grab toys from other children

- observe other children playing with the toy they want, but do not have strategies to ask for a turn

- prefer to play by themselves or with an adult

- have difficulties with joining in with games appropriately, and therefore appear as withdrawn or aggressive.

Ways to encourage sharing in the later stages

💬 Ensure that children are regularly reminded about boundaries and that sharing is expected.

💬 During a play session you could comment on other children's ability to share equipment and toys successfully.

💬 Consider using a visual cue (eg a sand timer) to support the child to play for a limited time with a toy, which is then passed on to another child.

💬 Read stories to the whole class that illustrate good sharing.

💬 Set up activities where children have to share equipment (eg to create a piece of artwork together or build a model).

💬 Give the child choices instead of demanding that they share a specific toy (eg 'Sarah would like to play with some soft toys. Which ones would you like to let her play with?').

💬 In small groups play turn-taking games, praising the child when they wait for their turn or share toys.

💬 Ensure that you use specific and immediate praise (see Glossary) when you see the child doing 'good sharing'.

💬 Try putting children in pairs and giving them one activity (eg a puzzle) between them. Support them to take turns – this will help them to understand the advantages of reaching a common goal together.

💬 Ensure that the child has opportunities to observe other children sharing appropriately – use peer praise (praising other children in the group) to highlight the behaviours you would like to see.

💬 In circle time (see Glossary) activities encourage children in the group to say if they feel another child has demonstrated good sharing.

Speechmark 💬

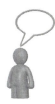

Social interaction

Why do we need to negotiate and make compromises?

As children become older, more complex social skills develop, such as the ability to negotiate and make compromises. These are important life skills that enable problem solving in many social situations. Children with social communication difficulties often need to be taught these skills explicitly.

Children who have difficulty with negotiation and compromise:

- may find it difficult to listen to and understand other children's points of view

- may have difficulties being aware of their own opinions and how these relate to others

- will often refuse to engage in conversations about negotiation (hold a 'black and white' view)

- may have difficulties with certain subjects or topics where they have to view something from somebody else's perspective (eg as in history, geography and religious education)

- may get into trouble both in and out of the classroom and be difficult to reason with

- may have difficulties maintaining friendships.

Ways to encourage negotiation and compromising skills

These skills are best practised within a group situation because the children will learn to listen to and understand what each wants, compare this with what they want themselves and find a way to meet halfway (compromise).

- Practise negotiation and compromise within a social skills group in which the children have to generate and adhere to the rules of their group.

- Consider using television footage from popular programmes, such as soap operas, demonstrating positive and poor examples of negotiation and compromise.

- Consider using video as a tool for self-reflection – use it as a pre- and post-analysis to show the children their progress.

- To give the children ownership of the group, encourage them to generate the topics they wish to focus on (within reason!).

- Within the group, work through scenarios (eg booking a restaurant). Encourage the children to assign themselves roles (eg phoning to book, finding out about public transport). Talk about problem solving what might go wrong.

- Discuss other issues for which the children are required to think about other people's points of view (eg vegetarianism, animal testing, school rules and current affairs).

- In groups, support members to experience negotiation and compromise through voting and majority rule (eg choosing a game to play or an activity to do after school).

Social interaction

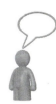

Why is it important to have friends?

The ability to make and maintain friendships and relationships is a key life skill. The function of friendship includes a sense of belonging within a community, adding meaning to life, happiness and contentment, support, security and companionship.

The ability to communicate effectively with others is essential in all aspects of life and especially in developing relationships and friendships. Children begin to learn these skills even from a very early age. Some children, however, need to be taught what is involved in friendships and also how to make and keep friends, as this does not always come naturally to them.

Children who have difficulty making friends may:

*   appear isolated in the classroom and playground

*   demonstrate play typical of younger children (eg cause-and-effect play, such as a noisy shape sorter) and are therefore not developmentally ready to engage in social- and interactive-type play

*   choose to play by themselves or stay with an adult, rather than interacting with their peers

*   initiate interaction with other children inappropriately (eg making silly noises or hugging them too aggressively)

*   have difficulties with joining in with group games appropriately, and therefore appear as withdrawn or aggressive.

89

Ways to encourage friendship skills in the early stages

💬 Ensure that there are opportunities for children to work in pairs, building up to small group work, supported by an adult.

💬 In paired play encourage the children to work together towards the same goal (eg building something together rather than being in competition with each other).

💬 Encourage the child to see what they have in common with other children (eg 'You both like playing with cars', 'You went to the same pre-school').

💬 Specifically praise (see Glossary) behaviour that is considered to be friendly (eg 'You're a good friend because you gave Jennifer one of your bricks').

💬 Try pairing children together in order to foster relationships – consider pairing a child with difficulties with a suitable role model.

💬 Encourage children to learn the names of other children through name games, such as 'I am Rolling the Ball to …' (support this using photos of children in the group).

💬 Sing group songs that encourage children to choose a friend or partner (eg 'The Farmer's in His Den').

💬 Ask children to choose a friend with whom to do an activity.

💬 Encourage the joining of clubs or activities that revolve around special interests for children outside nursery or school.

💬 Consider setting up a social skills group (see Glossary) to develop some early skills of interaction. See, for example, *Time To Talk* (Schroeder, 2001) or *The Social Use of Language Programme* (Rinaldi, 1995).

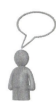

Social interaction

HOW TO ENCOURAGE THE DEVELOPMENT OF
FRIENDSHIP SKILLS – LATER STAGES

6i

Why do we need friendships?

The ability to make and maintain friendships and relationships is a key life skill. The function of friendship includes a sense of belonging within a community, adding meaning to life, happiness and contentment, support, security and companionship.

The ability to communicate effectively with others is essential in all aspects of life and especially in developing relationships and friendships. Children begin to learn these skills even from a very early age. Some children, however, need to be taught what friendships entail and also how to make and keep friends, as this does not always come naturally to them.

Children who have difficulty making friends:

- may appear isolated in the classroom and playground

- may initiate interaction with other children inappropriately (eg making silly noises or hugging them too aggressively)

- appear socially immature compared with their peers

- may seek out interaction with adults rather than with their peers or prefer to play with younger children

- may have difficulties with joining in with games and activities appropriately, and therefore may appear as aggressive or difficult

- may appear withdrawn or depressed

- can be the victims of bullying.

Ways to encourage friendship skills in the later stages

- Consider setting up a social skills group (see Glossary) or 'friendship group' where you explicitly teach what a friend is, how to meet and keep friends, how to greet friends and identification of what friends should and shouldn't do. It may be helpful to follow a published programme, such as *Socially Speaking* (Schroeder, 2000), *The Social Use of Language Programme* (Rinaldi, 1995), *Talkabout Activities* (Kelly, 2003) or *Talkabout Relationships* (Kelly, 2004)

- Set up a 'circle of friends' (see Glossary), in which socially able children have volunteered to support other children in developing relationships, or pair a child up with a suitable role model who can support that child's development of friendship skills.

- Consider setting up a 'friendship stop' in the playground, which is monitored by more able children. A 'friendship stop' is a specified place they can visit when they are feeling lonely. This will need to be carefully planned with the children who volunteer to help.

- Specifically praise (see Glossary) behaviour that is considered to be friendly (eg 'You're a good friend because you let Mark have the first go').

- Have discussions with children in the class about friendships, about how we are all different and about accepting or forming friendships with children despite their differences.

- Encourage the joining of clubs or activities that revolve around special interests for children outside nursery or school.

- Identify a specified place (such as a classroom) or member of staff where children can go if they are feeling lonely or isolated.

- Write Social Stories™ (Gray, 2001) to develop a child's understanding of how to make and maintain friendships.

- In structured activities allow children opportunities to practise joining in with a game, initiating a conversation and taking turns.

- Teach the qualities that make a good friend (eg shared interests, kindness, shared humour and shared experiences) and how to recognise that a friendship may not be genuine.

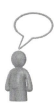

Social context

Why we need to adapt our style of communication for different social contexts

When communicating with different people it is usual to recognise the need to adapt our style of communication according to the situation or place we are in, the person we are talking to and the timing of our conversation. For example, we might talk quite casually and with humour to our good friends, be more reserved with strangers and more formal with people in authority. Style of communication is not just about the content of what we are saying, it is also about the way we say it (eg volume, tone of voice, posture and facial expression).

Children with social communication difficulties can find it difficult to understand different social contexts and may:

* lack awareness of how to approach people appropriately

* be over-familiar with adults and/or be too adult-like with peers

* be vulnerable in certain situations by not recognising boundaries, 'stranger danger' etc

* be overly tactile (eg not recognising that although it is appropriate to hug and kiss a parent, this is not appropriate with a teacher)

* alienate peers by being the 'voice of the teacher' in social situations

* find informal or unstructured activities difficult to deal with because they lack understanding of the unwritten rules.

Ways to teach children about different social contexts

💬 Explore with the children the ways in which styles of communication differ, with reference to both content and style (eg joking, teasing and being informal with friends, but being polite to teachers; speaking loudly in the playground, but quietly during religious observances; talking about their interests with people they know well, rather than starting a conversation with strangers at the bus stop).

💬 Practise the different ways to communicate through acting and role play and the use of some key phrases (eg demonstrate to the children the difference between the way to greet their peers and the way to greet adults).

💬 Play sorting games with phrases or actions written on pieces of paper, where the child has to decide what style of communication is appropriate to use with whom.

💬 Use conversation cue cards (see Glossary) to illustrate appropriate ways to initiate interaction in certain situations.

💬 Help the children to understand how their style of interaction is perceived by others.

💬 Use DVDs or television programmes to identify different ways of talking and practise these in drama sessions.

💬 Use Social Stories™ (Gray, 2001) or *Comic Strip Conversations* (Gray, 1994) to highlight inappropriate interaction in a particular situation and explore what would have been better in that situation.

💬 Use techniques such as 'circle of friends' (see Glossary) and 'Social Filing Cabinets' (Northumberland County Council Communication Support Service, 2004) to explore the varying degrees of familiarity of people in the child's life and ways to interact appropriately with those people.

Speechmark

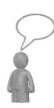

Understanding intentions

WORKSHEET 8A

What are the issues with bullying?

(The following suggestions are made specifically in relation to children with social communication difficulties and should be considered alongside the school bullying policy.)

Children with social communication difficulties are often a target of bullying for the following reasons:

- A frequent desire to be alone in the playground can single these children out as targets.

- They are often passive and will allow things to be taken from them.

- They can be quick to react in an emotional way.

- A lack of understanding of the unwritten codes of the playground (and who may or may not be a good person to know) makes these children socially vulnerable.

- They are also made vulnerable by a lack of conformity to social conventions (eg hobbies, interests, dress sense appropriate to peer group).

These children often lack an understanding of what bullying actually is and can over- or under-report incidents of bullying. Retaliation to a subtle bullying behaviour can result in them taking the blame. There can also be copying of 'bullying' behaviour without realisation of its consequences. Poor social understanding and the desire to have friends can leave a child with social communication difficulties vulnerable to being manipulated by others. The consequences of this can be significant.

Children who are being bullied may:

- show behaviours that are seen and reported by others

- show physical evidence (eg lost and damaged possessions or clothing, injuries)

- have increased anxiety (which can be shown in a number of ways)

- have their parents reporting school refusal

- show changes in their behaviour (becoming withdrawn or depressed)

- show an escalation of violent or disruptive behaviour or retaliation.

95

  Speechmark

WORKSHEET 8A

Ways to deal with bullying

Any attempts to deal with bullying should include all the people involved in the act (ie victim and perpetrator).

- Ensure that whatever the sanction is it should mean something to the individual child.

- Make the child who is being bullied aware both of 'safe havens' (see Glossary) around the school and of key members of staff; this can be done by creating a visual map of identified safe places and a list of names of members of staff and where they can be found that have been created in the school environment.

- Consider a buddy system or a 'circle of friends' (see Glossary) for playtimes and other unstructured times.

- Use Social Stories™ (Gray, 2001) to help change specific behaviours and *Comic Strip Conversations* (Gray, 1994) to look at misunderstandings and explore the range of responses and consequences.

- Teach about intention by exploring the difference between planned and unplanned (deliberate and accidental) events using role play, video, etc.

- Specifically teach (ie through a social skills group or individually) about the differences between passive, aggressive and assertive behaviours.

- Encourage open and frequent liaison between parents and school staff.

Speechmark

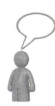

Understanding intentions

What are the issues with facts, lies and opinions in children with social communication difficulties?

A lack of ability to see things from another person's point of view can lead to difficulties with accepting others' opinions. Children with social communication difficulties usually find it impossible to tell lies, including white lies, as these involve the manipulation of someone else's thoughts. Therefore, even though they might understand that the consequences would be different if they lied, lying is just perceived to be illogical.

Lack of flexibility of thought can lead to these children learning something one way and finding it very difficult to accept that there can be other ways of understanding it or different meanings or interpretations of what is said. They can become upset when things they see as 'facts' are disputed by others.

Children who have difficulty distinguishing between facts, lies and opinions:

- can appear rude by telling the truth rather than using white lies or keeping quiet (ie commenting on someone's appearance, smell or actions negatively)

- can become distressed if lies are told and may find it difficult to allow peers to lie, without informing an adult

- can have difficulty accepting other people's opinions if those opinions are different from their own

- are socially vulnerable because they may not understand when they are being lied to by others.

Ways to develop an understanding of the function of facts, lies and opinions

💬 Organise a sorting activity with statements written on pieces of paper, to explore what is a 'fact' ('the table has four legs') and what is an opinion ('football is exciting').

💬 Explore different scenarios to look at intentions behind use of language (ie to deceive, to avoid hurting someone's feelings, etc).

💬 Use stories to explore characters' intentions.

💬 Discuss the potential and real consequences of lying.

💬 Use Social Stories™ (Gray, 2001) to explain the reasons for and consequences of lying and define the appropriate response.

💬 Teach stock phrases and questions to help the child to establish whether what is said is fact or opinion, true or not true.

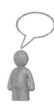

Understanding intentions

HOW TO ENCOURAGE THE UNDERSTANDING AND USE OF HUMOUR

8c

What are the issues with humour in children with social communication difficulties?

Understanding humour begins with an appreciation of slapstick and later evolves into verbal humour. Children with social communication difficulties do not lack a sense of humour; rather, they lack the knowledge and understanding of the intentions of others, of the multiple meanings of words and of social conventions, and are unlikely to be amused by the unpredictable. They also tend to make literal interpretations of what is said to them and they may therefore have difficulty with word-play jokes or puns (eg 'Why do barbers make good drivers? Because they know all the short cuts').

Many social relationships are supported by a shared sense of humour – difficulties in this area therefore have a huge impact on social integration.

Children who have difficulty with humour may:

- learn a joke in the playground that has resulted in others' laughter, but not realise the inappropriateness of using it in other contexts

- find things funny that are not obvious to others and can laugh out loud at inappropriate moments or with some delay

- not appreciate practical jokes, but only the breaking of rules involved

- have difficulties with understanding facial expression and tone of voice in humour, which may lead to difficulties with sarcasm

- be upset when people find some of the things they say and do funny when they had not intended them to be.

TOURO COLLEGE LIBRARY

Ways to develop an understanding of humour

● Explain the social purpose of jokes and humour, and how it is shared.

● Explore specific jokes and together work out why they are funny (eg explore play on words, unexpected events and what constitutes 'silliness').

● Teach different types of jokes and why they are funny.

● Encourage the child to notice and record what makes others laugh and to compare these with what makes them laugh.

● Explain to the child, and the class, that humour is personal and individual and that it is OK not to laugh if they don't find things funny.

Selecting and Organising Information

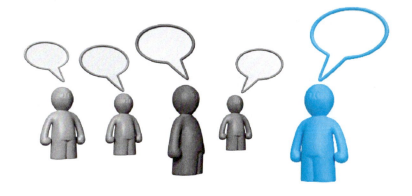

Listener needs

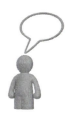

WORKSHEET 9A

What do we mean by listener needs?

In order for communication to be successful, the speaker needs to be aware of what the listener does and does not know about the subject. It is typical for very young children to assume that their listener knows what they know (eg if talking about an event, they will assume the listener knows where they were, who they were with, that they have a sister, and so on). As they grow older they understand that they need to provide the listener with more information and to give a clear context. Children with social communication difficulties are slower in developing these skills and some may never fully achieve them.

Children who have difficulty understanding listener needs:

- may give detailed information about specific things without first providing the 'bigger picture'

- may use general words, such as 'he', 'she' or 'their', without referring to the name of a person or place first

- are often unaware of how their topic may be uninteresting to others

- may have difficulty answering questions that are too general or vague (eg 'What did you do at school today?' as opposed to 'Did you have PE today?')

- may have difficulty providing an organised framework for information (eg they may not talk about events in a sequential order or they may talk about parts of a subject for a disproportionate length of time – 'going off at a tangent')

- may become frustrated by their perception of others' stupidity or may not understand others' frustration.

Ways to teach children about listener needs

Be specific in your feedback about where a breakdown in communication occurs, and why. Flag up your needs as a listener by asking questions to clarify when the context is not given.

Play games such as Give Us a Clue (see Glossary) or Pictionary (Mattel), which require the player to give the main points verbally or in drawings.

Encourage the child to think about a framework for giving information (eg who? where? when?) as background at the beginning. Practise these skills with cue cards and story planners.

Teach about others' interests and opinions in order to develop an understanding that we don't all feel the same or have the same interests and knowledge.

Use role play or video to demonstrate effective awareness of listener needs.

Use Social Stories™ (Gray, 2001) to explain the need to give the context to the listener and how the listener feels if this doesn't happen.

Teach about recognising signs that show that a listener is confused or bored, and key phrases and questions to check this (eg 'Do you understand?').

Play barrier games (see Glossary) (eg making a model or a drawing) to help develop an understanding of listener needs.

Speechmark

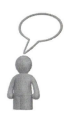

Narrative skills

9b

WORKSHEET 9B

What are narrative skills?

Narrative skills are the ability to tell a story – this may be spoken or written and may include:

- retelling a favourite story
- describing a television programme, a film or a play
- explaining something that has happened in the child's day (eg at playtime)
- telling news from the weekend
- making up new stories.

The Black Sheep Press 'Narrative' programmes (Black Sheep Press *et al*, 2001) list five key components that are needed when telling a story. That is, the child needs to describe:

- **who** was there
- **where** it happened
- **when** it happened
- **what** happened
- **the end** or the outcome.

Children who have difficulty with their narrative skills:

- may find it hard to start and finish stories appropriately

- may leave out crucial information or key points when telling a story

- find it difficult to expand on ideas and answer questions fully

- find it difficult to link elements and sequence information so that the story flows

- find it difficult to use appropriate grammar and sentence formation to link ideas (eg using 'and' and 'because')

- may assume that the listener shares their knowledge (eg referring to 'he' or 'she' and assuming that the listener knows who 'he' or 'she' is)

- may have a limited vocabulary or word finding difficulty, which can impact on their ability to use language creatively.

105

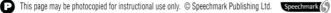

Ways to help children improve their narrative skills in the early stages

- Develop vocabulary skills by reading with children and allowing them to access a range of experiences from which they will learn new words.

- Repeat new words over and over and in different contexts (a child needs to hear a word many times before they can say it themselves).

- Develop listening skills by teaching children rules of good listening. Carry out small group work in which children have to learn to wait and take turns, and play games involving listening to sounds or words.

- Read stories, use story sacks (see Glossary), sing nursery rhymes and ask questions about these, focusing on the narrative framework
(eg ask '**Who** was in the story?', '**Where** were they?'). Focus on one component at a time
(eg 'Who?'). You may need to prime the children for what to listen for (eg 'I'm going to tell you a story and I want you to listen for **who** is in it').

- Act out stories and nursery rhymes, encouraging dressing up as characters.

- Incorporate narrative into day-to-day events (eg talking about '**Who** is here today?' or '**Where** is …?'). Use Makaton signs (see Glossary) and visual cue cards (see Glossary) when you talk about each of the narrative elements (eg who, where, when, what happened, the end).

- Follow the *Speaking and Listening through Narrative* programmes as published by Black Sheep Press *et al* (2001).

Speechmark

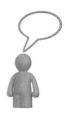

Narrative skills

WORKSHEET 9C

What do we mean by listener needs?

Narrative skills are the ability to tell a story – this may be spoken or written and may include:

- retelling a favourite story
- describing a television programme, a film or a play
- explaining something that has happened in the child's day (eg at playtime)
- telling news from the weekend
- making up new stories.

The Black Sheep Press 'Narrative' programmes (Black Sheep Press *et al*, 2001) list five key components that are needed when telling a story. That is, the child needs to describe:

- **who** was there
- **where** it happened
- **when** it happened
- **what** happened
- **the end** or the outcome.

Children who have difficulty with their narrative skills:

- may find it hard to start and finish stories appropriately
- may leave out crucial information or key points when telling a story
- find it difficult to expand on ideas and answer questions fully
- find it difficult to link elements and sequence information so that the story flows
- find it difficult to use appropriate grammar and sentence formation to link ideas (eg using 'and' and 'because')
- may assume that the listener shares their knowledge (eg referring to 'he' or 'she' and assuming that the listener knows who 'he' or 'she' is)
- may have a limited vocabulary or word finding difficulty, which can impact on their ability to use language creatively.

Speechmark

Ways to help children improve their narrative skills in the later stages

💬 Talk about stories, comic strips, films and television programmes. Discuss narrative components (eg who was in it, where it took place).

💬 Use a narrative framework to help children discuss their news with the class.

💬 Encourage children to make up a story either individually or in groups. Ask them first to think about each narrative component (eg '**Who** is going to be in your story?', '**Where** will it take place?') and then encourage them to use this structure to write or narrate their story.

💬 Use picture cards representing each of the narrative elements (ie different characters for '**who**' and different places for '**where**'). The children pick cards at random and make up a story containing these elements.

💬 Explicitly teach traditional story starters (eg 'Once upon a time …') and finishers ('And they lived happily ever after').

💬 Tell stories in which a component of narrative is missing (eg use 'he' or 'she' but don't explain who 'he' or 'she' is and see whether the children can identify what was missing and what the problems are with this).

💬 Follow the *Speaking and Listening through Narrative* programmes (Black Sheep Press *et al*, 2001).

💬 Use Makaton signs (see Glossary) and visual cue cards (see Glossary) when you talk about each of the narrative elements (eg who, where, when, what happened, the end). A bookmark or sheet containing the narrative structures can be a useful reminder for children when listening, reading or writing.

Speechmark 🟢

Sequencing

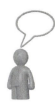

HOW TO ENCOURAGE THE UNDERSTANDING OF **SEQUENCING**

Why is it important to understand sequencing?

We use sequencing skills to understand why and how ideas fit together. This understanding is important in helping us to predict outcomes. If we do not recognise that events follow a logical sequence, we cannot anticipate how those events will end. The ability to sequence ideas, thoughts and pictures supports all of our learning.

We use the language of sequencing (eg 'first', 'before, after' and 'next') in many different aspects of learning. These concepts are crucial in subjects such as numeracy and literacy.

Children who have difficulty understanding and following sequences may:

- not be able to follow instructions in the correct order

- struggle to understand cause-and-effect relationships

- not be able to tell a story or recall events in a logical order, both verbally and in their writing

- struggle to understand concepts of time (eg days of the week)

- find it difficult to follow or remember simple routines (eg regular classroom activities)

- find it hard to predict outcomes of events.

WORKSHEET 9D

Ways to help children understand and follow sequences

Teaching children how to sequence, be it visually, verbally or in their writing, can help them learn to make appropriate predictions. It can also help them to have a better understanding of the relationship between individual events.

- Start with two or three pictures of situations a child has experienced and build on these, using 'Colorcards' sequencing cards (available from Speechmark Publications) to help the child begin to identify simple and familiar sequences – leave the last card out and see whether the child can describe what might happen next.

- Use cut-up pictures from familiar stories or simple sequencing pictures and ask the children to organise these so that the story makes sense.

- Encourage the children to guess outcomes during subjects such as science.

- Role play simple routines (eg getting up in the morning) with discussion about why things are done in a certain order. Reinforce this with visual support (eg a visual timetable).

- Use books to discuss sequences of events and discuss what might happen next.

- Use storytelling or writing to encourage sequencing of ideas in a logical manner.

Glossary

Barrier games

Two people sit either side of a barrier; one gives verbal instructions to carry out a task (eg describing a picture), which the other carries out without visual support. When the barrier is removed the two pictures should look the same.

Buddy system

Where a child with social communication difficulties is paired with a more socially able child to help foster friendship skills.

Circle of friends

Where socially able children have volunteered to support other, less able children in developing relationships.

Circle time games

Games used in schools during Personal, Social and Health Education to encourage development of personal and social skills. Resources can usually be found in schools.

Communication passport

A booklet all about the strengths and needs of individual children, and useful strategies they can use, which is shared with the adults working with those children.

Conversation cue cards

A system of simple, written resources (eg a list of different greetings) designed to provide a prompt for conversation skills.

'Give Us a Clue' games

Games (eg 'Twenty Questions') in which a child has to ask questions or give information in order to guess a target word or object.

Group eye contact games

Games, such as 'Wink Murder' and 'Pass the Look', in which children are encouraged to make eye contact with each other.

Makaton

A system of communication for people with communication and/or learning difficulties, which uses manual signs, graphic symbols and speech – visit the website www.makaton.org for more details.

Model

Show the desired behaviour or language by using it yourself for the child to see. This does not mean that the child needs to copy your language or behaviour.

Narrative skills

The skills of telling a story in a logical, relevant way, using key elements (eg who, when, where, what happened).

Narrative cue cards

Colour coded cards with a written word and symbol on to represent story elements such as who? where? when? and what happened?

'Pass the Expression'

Children sit in a circle and pass a specific expression (eg a sad face) to the person sitting next to them.

Reward chart

A chart on which a child can put stickers or tokens that he/she earns. A visual system for the child to keep track of his/her successes and rewards.

Reward system

This can be a token system, the opportunity for choosing a preferred activity or simply playing a game at the end of a task. Ideally, it should be visually represented (eg by stickers) to give children a clear understanding of what they are working towards.

Sabotage

Manipulating a situation in order to create a communication opportunity (eg not giving out paintbrushes during a painting activity so children have to ask for one).

Safe havens

Designated places within school where a child can go to feel 'safe'.

Social skills group

A group designed to develop children's social communication skills during short, structured activities. A number of published packages are available: see References.

Social stories

Simple, picture-based stories designed to help a child understand the consequences of their actions and help them learn desired behaviours. Further reading can be found in the References.

Specific praise

Explicitly stating the action that prompted the praise (eg rather than saying 'Good boy' or 'Good girl', you might say 'That's good sitting, well done').

Story sacks

A bag containing a story book and related props, models and activities.

Theory of mind

A term used to describe a person's awareness of their own mental process (eg their beliefs, intentions or knowledge) and the mental processes of other people.

Visual prompts/cue cards

A system of picture- or symbol-based resources designed to provide a tangible prompt for specific behaviours (eg a picture of an ear to prompt good listening).

References

Black Sheep Press with Stockport NHS Trust & Stockport PCT (2001)
Speaking and Listening through Narrative, Black Sheep Press, Keighley.

Frost L & Bondy A (2002) *The Picture Exchange Communication System*, Pyramid Educational Products Inc., USA.

Gaetano JG (1996) *Problem Solving Activities*, Great Ideas for Teaching Inc., Wrightsville Beach, NC, USA.

Gray C (1994) *Comic Strip Conversations: Colourful Illustrated Interactions with Students with Autism and Related Disorders*, Future Horizons, TX, USA.

Gray C (2001) *The New Social Stories Book*, Future Horizons, TX, USA.

Kelly A (1997) *Talkabout: A Social Communication Skills Package*, Speechmark Publishing, Milton Keynes.

Kelly A (2003) *Talkabout Activities: Developing Social Communication Skills*, Speechmark Publications, Milton Keynes.

Kelly A (2004) *Talkabout Relationships: Building Self-Esteem and Relationship Skills*, Speechmark Publications, Milton Keynes.

Martin L (1990) *Think It – Say It: Improving Reasoning and Organisation Skills*, Communication Skill Builders, supplied by Winslow Press, Bicester.

Northumberland County Council Communication Support Service (2004) *Autistic Spectrum Disorders: Practical Strategies for Teachers and Other Professionals*, David Fulton Publishers, London.

Phillips N & Beavan L (2007) *Teaching Play to Children with Autism: Practical Interventions using Identiplay*, Lucky Duck Publishers, London.

Rinaldi W (1995) *The Social Use of Language Programme (Primary and Pre-school Teaching Pack)*, Windsor, NFER.

Rippon H (2005) *Think About It*, Black Sheep Press, Keighley.

Rippon H, **Black Sheep Press with Stockport PCT & Stockport MBC** (2002) *Nursery Narrative Pack*, Black Sheep Press, Keighley.

Schroeder A (2000) *Socially Speaking: A Pragmatic Social Skills Programme for Primary Pupils*, LDA, Cheshire.

Schroeder A (2001) *Time To Talk: A Programme to Develop Social Interaction Skills at Reception and Key Stage One*, LDA, Cheshire.

Speechmark